the
power of
tranquility
in a
very noisy
world

the power of tranquility in a very noisy world

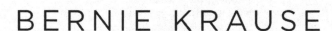

BERNIE KRAUSE

Little, Brown and Company

New York Boston London

Little, Brown and Company
Hachette Book Group
1290 Avenue of the Americas, New York, NY 10104

littlebrown.com

First Edition September 2021

Little, Brown and Company is a division of Hachette Book Group, Inc. The Little, Brown name and logo are trademarks of Hachette Book Group, Inc.

The publisher is not responsible for websites (or their content) that are not owned by the publisher.

The Hachette Speakers Bureau provides a wide range of authors for speaking events. To find out more, go to hachettespeakersbureau.com or call (866) 376-6591.

Photo credit p.125: Katherine Krause, © 2021 Wild Sanctuary. All rights reserved.

ISBN 978-0316-42106-5

Library of Congress Control Number: 2021940976

Printing 1, 2021

LSC-C

Printed in the United States of America

*To Al Young
and the memory of
Stuart Gage*

Contents

the
power of
tranquility
in a
very noisy
world

Introduction

"What is essential is invisible to the eye."
Antoine de Saint-Exupéry, *The Little Prince*

The closest I've come to an authentic holy rendez-vous was on a gentle October afternoon more than half a century ago. I had gone alone to a small sub-urban park just north of San Francisco. My mission that day was nothing special. It was simply to record natural sounds for an album my late music partner, Paul Beaver, and I were creating for Warner Bros. The album, *In a Wild Sanctuary,* was to be the first of its kind dedicated to the theme of ecology, and also the first to incorporate entire soundscapes—urban and natural—mixed as components of the orchestration. That moment was also my first attempt to record sound outdoors.

As luck would have it, portable stereo tape recorders had just been introduced and Paul and I had been given one of the early models to experiment with. I knew nothing about recording outside and was, frankly, a bit unnerved about what dangers I might encounter, even in a carefully managed public park replete with well-marked trails and signage. All of my sound work to that moment had been from an interior perspective—studios or film sound stages— places mostly without windows or connections to the earthly world beyond. It had never crossed my mind that there was another domain that could offer so much gratification, so many thrilling encounters, so much splendor and, moreover, a remedy for my lifelong affliction with ADHD. These feelings, mostly unexpressed in the insulated childhood biome where I spent my early years and in the places I would later work as a young adult, were freighted at that instant of recognition with a measure of uncertainty and trepidation. But by midafternoon on that fall day, the trajectory of my life had already changed.

In the late sixties, most fall off-season weekdays in the park drew very few visitors. There were certainly none in sight where I had set up to record. I was alone with no distractions. Standing by a small stream in the dappled shade of the redwood trees, listening to the soundscape through my earphones, I was immediately struck by an overwhelming impression of sanctity so unexpected and emotionally powerful that it almost brought me to tears. It wasn't completely quiet—true silence (or no sound) in the living world is rarely, if ever, encountered. A slight autumn breeze wafting through the forest canopy from the ocean just to the west combined with the soft trickle of water from a nearby stream made me feel calm for the first time that day. A pair of ravens passed overhead, the edge tones of their wingbeats marking a course through the sky above as the birds soared off into the distance. Every acoustic element enhanced the vast illusion of space transmitted through my new headphones. There certainly was sound. But what was it about those particular resonances that caused such an intense effect unknown to me before? For one thing, the noises that always made me feel on edge and wary in the city were nearly inaudible except for remote traces of park construction off in the distance. Mostly, though, I had found for myself a measure of tranquility—the kind that set in motion a direction and appeal I would follow for the rest of my time on this planet.

Before that event, the noise in my life had been a constant din of acoustic distraction, an unhealthy condition magnified by my ADHD and consequential hypersensitivity to noise of any kind. Yet, I was drawn to noise, like a moth to a flame, for the same reason any of us are seduced — because it creates the allure of action, curiosity, competition, and pursuit of the tenuous that I, and too many of us, cannot seem to live without.

Because of poor eyesight, my life has always been primarily informed by what I hear. From the time I first saw a picture of a recording studio when I was four or five, my goal was to become a professional musician. I had a violin in my hands by the time I was three and a half. At four, my violin teacher introduced me to composition. By thirteen, although I showed some promise, I became bored and switched to guitar, learning all styles thinking I would be able to study at college level. Then I got the first of many big life surprises: When I applied to Juilliard, Eastman School of Music, and the music department of the University of Michigan in 1955,

I was informed that the guitar was not a musical instrument.* After earning a degree in Latin American history, I went east and began to work in the early 1960s folk music scene around Boston. At one point, I was invited to audition for the tenor position in the well-known folk group the Weavers, the spot originated by the late Pete Seeger. I joined them for their last year together in 1963. After the Weavers broke up, I came to California to audit electronic music classes at Mills College in Oakland with Pauline Oliveros as my mentor, and attended lectures given by Karlheinz Stockhausen. There, I was introduced to Paul Beaver and together we formed the synth team Beaver & Krause. In 1967, we introduced the synthesizer to pop music and film, first at the Monterey Pop Festival, and then during a weekly series of workshops at Paul's studio in Los Angeles. We made five albums together; one of them charted. Until Paul's death we worked, individually or together, on more than a hundred major feature films, including *Rosemary's Baby, A Man Called*

---

* The guitar was not taught in any American music department until 1962, when it was introduced at Berklee College of Music, Boston.

Horse, The Illustrated Man, Love Story, Performance, Castaway, and *Apocalypse Now.* Artists we worked with included Mick Jagger, George Harrison, Van Morrison, the Doors, David Byrne, the Beach Boys, Linda Ronstadt, Brian Eno, and many others. In my role as a professional musician, it was, at first, fun to play endless sessions for major feature films and with influential artists and groups. Ego gratification is built on a foundation of noise, and, in the end, it came at a high price, ultimately making me sick. On my last major film session, after being fired more than half a dozen times while working on *Apocalypse Now,* where my task had been to generate the helicopter sounds and to program settings for about a third of the synthesized score, I quit music, went back to school, earned a PhD in creative sound arts with an internship in marine bioacoustics, and never looked back. I've spent the past half century capturing wild soundscapes in some of the most remote places on Earth, wherever life-affirming environments still thrived. In the process I have drawn on those blissful moments to learn the value of serenity, how to avoid the serious physical and emotional consequences of noise, and how to discover the acoustic environments that have a palliative effect on stress and anxiety. Our bodies know when things are right.

The Power of Tranquility in a Very Noisy World revisits that journey. Bit by bit we will discover what each one of us can do to realize the healing powers of positive acoustic encounters while, at the same time, reducing or eliminating the effects of the toxic sonic habitats that most of us find ourselves surrounded by. I'll explore with you the difference between harmful noise and the signals that make us feel good, between noise as a stressor and sound-scapes that serve as an emotional and physiological naturopath and productivity stimulator. By book's end you will have been introduced to techniques for eliminating unhealthy sounds in favor of restorative signals to be found primarily in natural world settings, ancient protosymphonies that are being revisited for their healing properties—some in your own neighborhoods—in effect, yoga for the ear.

But first, it's important to unravel the distinctions between noise, and therapeutic resonance. We'll do that through short forays into the environments where we all live. Follow these easy suggestions and you'll discover what a wide variety of sound signatures represent; which ones you like, which ones you don't, and why. Think of the first chapters as a kind of ear-arousal, a form of sonic Rosetta Stone on the one hand, and acoustic sanitizing exercises to help you reengage as we were originally meant to listen to the world on the other. Then, I'll explain the toxic effects of noise in our environments, what produces them, and what, individually and collectively, we can do about it. Finally, we'll embrace the kinds of acoustic decisions that transform our lives into nourishing, vibrant adventures.

People often ask, "If I want that more tranquil life you speak of, what can I do?" It's not what we have to do to reach this state of tranquility. It's what we *don't* do.

CHAPTER 1

Sound vs. Noise:

Clarity, at last.

⟞⟨⟞

"I doubt we will ever be able to 'listen' to our enemies or cause them to listen to us until we can hear our own noise with their ears."

Garret Keizer, *The Unwanted Sound of Everything We Want: A Book About Noise*

To paraphrase the late David Bowie, "The future belongs to those who can hear it coming." To hear it coming, though, we'll need to make some changes in the ways we listen. If I were to create a generalized acoustic portrait of myself and our younger friends and family, it might go something like this: We're everywhere. And so is all the sound that we manage to generate. In more normal times, we drift down city streets, over school grounds, parks, malls, and clubs. We rock earbuds or headphones, our noses buried in our smartphones, no notice paid to others or what else exists in the rich surroundings through which we pass. We seldom glance up. What for? We're held in thrall by the sounds of our e-world distractions, which, as of this writing include Spotify, Pandora, TuneIn, ringtones, Bandcamp, and gaming sounds, expanding exponentially in a Möbius strip mix list of constant reinvention. Our sonic ecosystem is crammed with hip-hop, country, rock, jazz. Lil Nas X, Mahler, Nicki Minaj, AC/DC. Music is everywhere and loud, mixed in and competing with everything else. We tune to whatever we *think* we want to listen to. But how much of it do we really *hear*?

When we don't have earbuds jammed into our ears, we're inundated with other noises. Older subways in our large cities produce an aggressive range of ear-splitting sound as metal grinds upon metal. The wrathful fury of straight-piping muscle cars and snarling motorcycles as they tear through our neighborhoods startle and frighten, precisely as they're meant to do. A TV program in another room adds to the acoustic mind clutter with lots of unintelligible acoustic debris. The din in restaurants where we eat and the streets we walk makes it difficult to enjoy our hard-earned nights out in peace, assuming we can go out at all in the midst of a pandemic. During an average weekday, jackhammers and the unrestrained jangle of construction sites make it impossible to relax, each sound-generating implement destined to distract and unsettle us physically and emotionally.

For the past two-and-a-half centuries, our lives have been increasingly beset by human noise. Yet, this distinctive class of sound has become so much of a part of our everyday experience that we've become oblivious to the damage it does to our hearing, our physical well-being, and our emotional health. During the early years of Airbnb my dear wife Kat and I rented out our Wild Sanctuary guesthouse. Located in Northern California on ten acres of an extended wildlife corridor, it served as an occasional bed-and-breakfast. One late summer weekend, a young couple from New York checked in for three nights. The morning after their arrival, when I left the house for my usual dawn run, the two of them were at the bottom of the stairs loading luggage into the trunk of their rental car. When I asked what was wrong, they said that the nighttime cricket sounds from the woods surrounding our place were terrifying and that they had decided to move into a downtown San Francisco hotel where they could hear the familiar sounds of the city. Young as they were, it was too late: The urban damage had already occurred.

If your ears are ringing after leaving a concert or a party because of the loud environment, the likelihood is that you've physically damaged your hearing. If the exposure has been for too long a period, some loss may be permanent. And for millennials, this is particularly notable: According to a 2017 article in *The Lancet,* one of the oldest and most reliable peer-reviewed publications on medical issues, hearing loss of the kind I've described is also "the largest modifiable risk factor for developing dementia, exceeding that of smoking, high blood pressure, lack of exercise and social isolation."[*]

At the same time, all too many of us have become oblivious to the nurturing sounds that these signals have supplanted. That's not surprising, because more and more, we're starved of them. Sounds like the rustle of leaves from a whisper of wind in the canopy of the trees above, a spring dawn or evening chorus,

[*] thelancet.com/commissions/dementia2017.

the gentle cooing of a mourning dove, or the amazing expressive range of crow vocalizations. Crashing waves at the ocean shore, the pulsing edge tones of a bird's wings as it navigates the airspace above us, the burst of hundreds of European starlings taking off all at once and diving in great murmurations over a winter wheat field all complement our sense of sonic wonder.

Some found the sudden fall in the clamor resulting from the COVID-19 virus isolation mandates disturbing. If that was the case for you, it might be an indication of just how much you've become habituated to noise. For me, that moment served as a respite from the intruding din that constantly distracts us.

From the accounts in this book, I hope you'll come to realize that we're not only missing so much of what's happening beyond the EarPods in our ears, but also the visual screen noise coming from your digital device puts you at a higher risk of getting hurt, thwacked by a car, running into others or a tree because we're so addicted and otherwise preoccupied at the same time. We're screwing up our ears and lives with all kinds of noise. So, what can we do about this problem?

At this point, let's revisit some old terms that have been misunderstood. As an exercise, several of my colleagues and I recently began to reevaluate soundscapes to see if they might contain important pieces of information we'd missed upon first hearing. To parse out those pieces, we began with the most obvious question: What's the difference between sound and noise?

Typically, the question has been answered this way: All sound is noise and all noise is sound. The late John Cage classified noise as undifferentiated sound. Question is, undifferentiated to whom? My coworkers and I have found that each type of sonic vibration has a different effect on us as well as on other living organisms. Music that you love elicits one kind of response. But the music you love might come across as "undifferentiated" to your partner or neighbor. Does that make it "noise"? A low-flying helicopter passing over your house on an otherwise quiet summer's night waking you from a deep, restful sleep contains no useful information to you. It's not quite undifferentiated sound, either, because you recognize the source. But it's still a type of noise that has an effect. Once you become conscious of what those effects are, you'll be able to decide which sources are useful and which ones you'll want to eliminate.

If we want healthy outcomes from our soundscapes, we must all learn to listen to the ways in which sound is organized—or not. Each of us thinks we're good listeners, and we get offended when someone tells us we're not listening to them. But in that case, we're not listening for *meaning:* we're listening for *meaningfulness,* or importance. A sound is important to us if it stimulates awareness or enjoyment. That makes it useful.

Psychologically, each of us can readily distinguish between the two types of signal that sound conveys. To be fair, noise is, indeed, made up of vibrations that comprise sound. And some sound *is* noise. In some quarters, noise has been defined as unwanted sound. That is certainly true. But there are some simple ways to clear up this otherwise noisy issue if we identify what we're actively listening for.

Beneficial sound vibrations contain valuable information. These I categorize as coherent sounds that carry messages most of us will want to pay some attention to. Language and music of the types we're familiar with fit into this category. So do the narratives coming from the stage in a theater, broadcasts from various media, a podcast of interest, or even announcements at an airport.

Then there are my favorite types of sound, those that spring bioacoustically from relatively undisturbed wild habitats. They include all the non-domestic

17

organisms that express themselves in the wild land- and seascapes of the world—the sounds produced by insects, reptiles, amphibians, birds, fishes, and mammals, among others. To those of us who have learned to listen, the knowledge contained in those narratives of place reveals just how dynamic a habitat can be. I think of these expressions as the earliest epic poems, in this case those of the natural world.

Then there are those random signals that to our ears are chaotic or incoherent; they contain no useful information at the time they're transmitted. They're distracting. I place these signals in the category of noise. I also think of noise as any disrupting sound that, in a given context, contains irrelevant or distorted transmissions coming mostly from human-made sources, usually from electronic or mechanical technologies. Think of static from a distant radio station, the whirr of the compressor in your fridge when it switches on, or the background hum of a CPU on the floor underneath the desk where your computer keyboard is located.

Typically, the noise I'm referring to doesn't need to be particularly loud; it's simply made of acoustic vibrations that distract us or make us uncomfortable. It could be a drone aircraft flying low over your living or working space. The drone may not be loud but the nature of its sound may distract you or cause alarm. A muscle car with windows rolled down and 808 speakers booming as it passes by your home on an otherwise quiet summer night could be equally disturbing for different reasons. A neighbor's sound system tuned to a sporting event and cranked so loud that you can't sleep with your bedroom windows open *or* closed. Maybe the noise comes from a backyard party down the street. Doesn't matter; lose a few good nights' sleep because of noise and you'll be at risk for all kinds of adverse physical and psychological consequences.

But how do we describe the total sonic fabric of our daily lives?

Everything we take in visually outdoors, whether urban, rural, or wild, represents a landscape, cityscape, or seascape. In the same way, the collective sound we hear from all the various sources that reach our ears at a given moment is referred to as the soundscape, whether it's indoors or out. If we break these acoustic entities down into their various parts, we find that each soundscape is made of different vibrating sources produced within our field of hearing. All in all, there are three basic types of sources that contribute to this sonic fabric. One or more will be present in any given soundscape.

The first strand that makes up the texture of the soundscape is the *geophony*. This source is composed of nonbiological natural sounds like the effects of wind in the forest canopy of trees or wafting through low-lying grasses; water in a stream, gentle or torrential rain, volcanoes, earthquakes, firestorms, avalanches. Present for the entire lifespan of the earth—about 4.5 billlion years—these geophonies are the oldest known sounds the planet has produced. But there was nothing to hear these first signals until sound-sensitive organisms evolved around 550 million years ago. *Biophony,* the name given to this second category, consists of the collective sound produced by all nonhuman organisms in a given habitat at one period of time. (I factor humans out of this category because of our profound cultural disconnect to the natural world. While some sounds we produce may be considered biophonic, most of the sound we create now fits neatly into a class all its own. Read on.) And, finally, our own recent contribution to the sonic tapestry that first appeared roughly two million years ago is called the *anthropophony:* human-generated sound. Let's not forget that the most significant impact of anthropophony has been felt within the last 250 years beginning with the Industrial Revolution. Anthropophony is divided into two sub-categories: intentionally controlled sound such as music, theater, and spoken word performances, and sound installations; and chaotic, random or incoherent sounds referred to earlier, mostly generated by our electromechanical devices, the primary sources of human noise.

To understand these features better, take a moment to imagine your own immediate acoustic environment. Think of the typical sound field most of us are immersed in as a pyramid. I imagine the bottom of the mass as filled with murky signals with this segment representing all of the combined sounds and noises you're likely to encounter in urban and many rural environments, the habitats where most of us live. The stages in between are populated with various mixes of competing sound with each elevated layer featuring increased nourishing acoustic energy until we get to the top segment, the one that represents the healthiest sonic environment, tranquility. I'll talk more about this ultimate grouping in the last chapters.

Try this: Leave your smartphone in the house for a few minutes, grab a piece of paper and a pen, and step outside. You don't have to go too far; just out the front door of your house or apartment building will do. Take a moment to listen carefully to the sounds around you. If you live in a city or rural area, note that different types of vehicles produce unique kinds of sound. Large, heavy trucks emit characteristic expressions; their transmissions and engines are designed to pull heavier loads, and their particular types of power sources produce acoustic signatures that can be quite loud. Lighter and smaller trucks or vans generate their own special sound marks. A motorcycle, modified with a set of straight exhaust pipes, produces a roar and crackle specifically designed to call attention to it— to momentarily distract you and every other living organism from what you're doing. Each type of aircraft signature is distinctive. During World War II, we lived not far from an air base. By the time I was six or seven years old, I could identify any type of aircraft flying over our house by the sound its engine produced. A small helicopter might sound like an irritating insect, while military or law enforcement choppers will sound ominous and formidable with a low-frequency *thump-thump* of the rotor cavitation that can be heard miles away over the right terrain and under the right atmospheric conditions. Corporate or commercial jet planes emit a range of sounds predicated in part on the type of aircraft, weather at your location, altitude, speed, and topography, and urban or rural structural or vegetation density. Commercial aircraft tend to be quieter than the military versions. Don't dismiss single-engine private aircraft, where each type radiates a unique signal. To the extent that your ears are still good, you have the capacity to distinguish all these sounds. But you may not normally listen to them. In fact, they're so common that in many of these cases you would tend to dismiss them entirely from your acoustic perception although those signals will affect you.

In the small-town neighborhood where Kat and I lived before the Northern California firestorms of 2017, late at night we might hear a dog barking in the distance, answered, in turn, by others in response. Two cats confronting each other in a nearby backyard hissing and yowling, posturing for territory. A train whistle off in the distance. Attempt to hear those performances at night. They can be magical.

In the city where you may live, and where the mechanical sound world dominates the mix of most natural acoustic textures, try to catch the song or call of birds and insects within that blend. Each of these sounds will have a different effect on you depending on the quality and context in which the signals are transmitted and received. Some sounds will be familiar. But listen more carefully and you'll almost always hear something new.

If you want to know generally how much noise there is in your neighborhood, try this: Record an American robin—the common bird with an orange-colored breast almost always vocalizing in the spring and summer months—with your smartphone. Listen to the playback. It will probably contain lots of other sounds that interfere with the birdsongs you're aiming to get. Try again. Not so good this time, either? Hint: It's likely that you'll need to get up way before sunrise to record the bird you want—a time when your neighborhood is still quiet. In the process of recording you'll begin to realize just how much intrusive noise there is in your environment.

In music, the special quality of an instrument's sound—like the difference in the acoustic characteristics between a trumpet and a violin—or the particular blend of many instruments performing at once is referred to as *timbre* (pronounced *tamber*). This concept is applicable to the broader, nonmusical sonic world as well. Timbre is important in natural and urban settings because it helps define for us a sense of place. For example, the timbre of a tropical rain forest sounds very different from that of temperate high deserts. New York at rush hour sounds very different from the small-town after-work ambience where we now live. The population here is just north of eleven thousand people. In a few words: At all hours, the ambience of small towns generally sounds more relaxed and laid back—a conditional story conveyed through the soundscape—and a reason why many people choose to live in those environments.

Another thing to think about: loud levels are not the only criterion for noises that are distracting or disturbing. The constant drip of a leaking faucet in your bathroom or kitchen could do it. If you are affected by certain noise types, like motorcycles, leaf blowers, or the constant muffled sound of your next-door neighbor's TV, even if they're not especially loud, these will eventually induce levels of stress and affect you physically. *Noise equals stress* is a simple equation. This is especially true for those of us who feel disturbed *and* powerless to control the acoustic source that induces the tension.

Before I focus on what to do about all this racket,

let's first consider the details contained in the composition of sound I've been discussing. Again, step outside your front door, close your eyes, and take in the soundscape that surrounds you. Alternatively, take a short sound walk—a leisurely jaunt around your neighborhood concentrating on just the sounds you hear. How many of the sounds you hear are natural, i.e., non-domestic birds, mammals, insects, or frogs? If you encounter stormy weather, do you hear the effects of wind blowing? Describe this to yourself. If it's raining, can you make out the sound of raindrops on the pavement or in the eaves of your house? If it's calm outside, can you describe the feeling of "calm"? From what you're hearing, how do all those sounds, together and individually, make you *feel*? Weather-wise, how would you differentiate a calm moment from a windy or stormy one? Describe the sound of snow falling. (Yes, it *does* create an acoustic signature.) And finally, a problem area we all share—human noise. Are you able to perceive the sources of all the different types of human-generated sound? When are these types of audio signals exciting to you? And, when are they not? Anyone can learn to do this, even if you're partially hearing impaired, as I became when I reached a certain age.

Take a moment to describe what you're hearing. Write them down so you can keep track of how your ability to parse out one signal from another improves over time. There are many ways to explain what we see because we're a visual culture. However, there are very few words to describe in detail what you hear. Make them up (for example, *geophony, biophony, anthropophony*). Listen, again, and note all of the noise sources. A command over these descriptions will help you to make good choices about your acoustic environments. First, however, some ideas to keep in mind regarding the sound walk or -listening break you just took.

Sound sources to consider: Given all of the sound sources you hear as you navigate through your daily environments and after your first sound walk, make a four-column list of sound sources, using the table below. One column is meant for those types you like, another for those that you don't. In the heading for the third column, you only need one word, "Why?" When you begin to consider the answer to these simple questions, a whole new world of experience opens up before you. In the fourth column, the question will be, "What will I do about it?"

Sound walk			
Sounds I Liked	Sounds I Didn't Like	Why?	What Will I Do About It?

CHAPTER 2

Physically Harmful Sounds:

Controlling the effects.

⸎

Now that you're aware of the structure of the soundscape and the differences between sound and noise, here's something about hearing that I'd like to share. Recently, our nephew and niece came by for a visit. They are tweens. Like most kids in their age group, nearly every waking minute their eyes were focused on their devices, gaming or texting away the hours, earbuds and screen images blocking contact with the rest of the living world around them. When I invited them to listen to some unusual animal sounds in my sound studio—their smartphones like safety blankets, never far out of reach—I had an opportunity to test their hearing by playing some high-frequency test sounds. Normally, young folks that age are able to hear nearly the full human range, including the upper end of the spectrum—somewhere between 18,000 and 20,000 hertz (hertz [or Hz] = frequency in cycles per second). I was blessed with being able to detect that range until I was seventy years old only because I was very sensitive to loud sound and protected my hearing from the time I was five or six. Given my lifelong encounters with ADHD, I paid some careful attention to safeguarding what I allowed my ears to encounter. But, according to my anecdotal test, it appeared that these youngsters had already lost more than 10 percent of their high-end bandwidth. (14kHz* was their upper limit, a staggering loss given their age.) At some point, these loss rates grow exponentially; at the rate they were going, it wouldn't be much longer before they might endure serious hearing impairment. They're not alone. For their peers, many in the same boat, that is not a good omen for a healthy outcome.

Despite these warnings, there are times when

---

* Fourteen thousand hertz

large crowds of all ages gather to take in the thrill of high-level noise events. Each October in San Francisco, the Blue Angels, the Navy's flight demonstration squadron, performs for throngs of more than a million people. In the pre-COVID era, crowds that lined the shores of the San Francisco Bay exceeded the city's actual population. The fly-bys and aerobatics are both electrifying and earsplitting, at times measured well above what's considered safe levels (85dB vs. 120dB).* In comparison, a rock concert in the 1970s (Motörhead) produced levels measured at 137.5dB, exceeding the Who's earlier record by 12dB, a factor of two. And on any given weekend during the summer months, racetracks, such as Sonoma Raceway just north of San Francisco, featured drag races and NASCAR events that delight 100,000 fans with extremely high levels of noise and where the spill of each event's low-frequency rumble can be heard and recorded at our home eighteen miles away! Ask any attendee at these gatherings why they come and they'll tell you that

---

* dB (decibel) is a measure of sound intensity sometimes commonly expressed as a single unit of change being the smallest variation that a human ear can detect.

they go for the thrill of power that the intense noise produces.

Speaking of noise and power, that reminds me of a comment made by James G. Watt, Ronald Reagan's secretary of the interior. Shortly after Watt defunded the US Office of Noise Abatement in 1982, a federal bureau that had played an important role in the Environmental Protection Agency, the bureau was left with no resources to enforce its safety mandates. When asked why he had targeted that group, Watt responded, "Noise is power. The noisier we are as Americans, the more powerful we appear to be to others."*

Then there are the noises of war and the despicable manner in which humans sometimes treat each other or members of other species with consequences too severe to rehash here. But there's one small incident worth noting because it amplifies Watt's distorted perspective on noise. In 2000, I was asked to give a presentation at a US Department of the Interior and National Park Service meeting in Washington, DC. The purpose of the meeting was

---

* R. Murray Schafer, *The Book of Noise,* Arcana Editions, 1998. Personal correspondence, March 2011.

to discuss how particular types of sound might be used to impact wildlife. One biologist, from the US Army's Aberdeen Proving Ground, described how cannon fire was being tested to see if it could successfully drive pesky birds away from the runways there. At the end of her presentation, the presenter was asked if the test was successful. "Not completely," she said, "but I love the sound of artillery. To me, it represents the sound of freedom." The room grew dead silent for a moment because no one knew quite what to say. Eager to break the ice, I raised my hand and asked, "But, Lieutenant, doesn't that depend on which side of the cannon you're standing?"

Frightening birds from airports with loud noise is an old trick that typically works only the first few times it's tried. Yet here's a curious application that resulted in a rather long-term effect: In 1999, the *Los Angeles Times* reported that rock diva Tina Turner's voice had been identified as an effective way to scare off birds hanging around the runways of England's Gloucestershire Airport, the landing field nearest the royal family's estates. Airport staff biologists had previously tried recordings of avian distress calls, other predators, and loud explosions to frighten the birds away from the runways but achieved only limited success. When they switched to loud recordings of the famed rock singer, there was an immediate and dramatic reduction in the number of birds that interfered with the landings and departures of corporate jets, helicopters, and other aircraft.*

For the record, the loudest sound in recent history didn't come from a rock concert or the battlefield. It came from the 1883 eruption of the Indonesian volcano Krakatoa. (It was estimated at 180dB, just 14dB short of the loudest physically possible sound on Earth.)† It was a geophonic explosion so loud that—depending on which historical account you read—it ruptured eardrums of people forty miles away, traveled around the world through the atmosphere four times as a physically sensed infrasound

---

* "Tina Turner Aversion," *San Francisco Chronicle*, September 19, 1999, where the article was syndicated.
† The loudest sustained sound on Earth's surface cannot possibly exceed 194dB—which is the point at which the amplitude of the sound wave is so intense that the low-pressure part is a perfect vacuum and where the wave alternates between double the normal atmospheric pressure and no air at all. No human being can survive a sound field that intense. Note: In water, a much denser medium, the maximum level is 270dB. Some whale species have produced estimated sound levels of around 200dB in their environments.

jolt and was clearly heard three thousand miles from the source. Humans have yet to match the extraordinary level of that blast. But the sounds we do create can be troublesome enough. Think, for a moment, of the loudest sound you've ever heard or the sound that was most disturbing.

Some of us try to block the noise around us by layering types of sounds we think we like on top. Even if we play the preferred sounds louder, that just adds confusion to the mix and we end up with competing signals, again. If you choose to do that, you still need to eliminate the competing signals within your range of hearing, or at least reduce them enough so that you're able to hear the sounds you do like. Even if all of us have headphones or earbuds designed to cut out rival sounds by adding others or noise-canceling, we're largely kidding ourselves. Mostly, we keep piling more conflicting information into our ears hoping to mask the debris we want to get rid of. We attempt this remedy by introducing levels of masking sound far louder than our sensitive organic hearing system can physically handle. At some point this becomes physically dangerous.

Is this a good strategy? Ask Pete Townshend, leader of one of history's great rock bands, the Who.

When he was young, his band's stack of 200-watt Marshall Major amps put out staggering levels of sound, and he loved it. So did his fans. He actually enjoyed the pain in his ears caused by the thrashing of guitars and drums—his way to physically bliss out on his music. But as he aged into his late twenties, he developed tinnitus—a nasty ringing in the ears and a consequence of early hearing loss brought on by exposure to loud performances. Many rock musicians suffer the same problem. There is no treatment. Lose your hearing to deafening sound and you're out of luck. It doesn't take much noise to damage hearing. And, once lost in that way, it cannot be restored.

You don't have to be a rock star to go deaf—far from it. Constant loud sound transmitted through earbuds or in environments where you work, live, drive, or play will do it. Way too many of my music friends became hearing impaired over a short period between the late 1960s and late 1980s. Most of us, as we age, lose some of the higher sounds in our range, anyway. In "Desperado," the Eagles sang, "You're losing all your highs and lows / Ain't it funny how the feeling goes away..." The Eagles may have been singing about moods. This could have also been a coded warning to their fans about our hearing. If so, listen up.

For those particularly sensitive to certain types of acoustic signals, here's a relatively new clinical condition to consider: It's a term called *misophonia*. (Same root word as in *misanthrope* and *misogyny*.) It refers to a condition in which ordinary signals such as a person chewing gum and generating a snapping noise with each bite, or breathing, fingers tapping, or even opening a plastic bag of chips become really irritating to the listener—actually making them angry. (Oprah will not allow anyone to chew gum in her presence.)

Getting back to our main theme, most critters that live within relatively undisturbed, vigorous habitats rely on some combination of their hearing, sight, ability to smell, touch, and the knack to process complex information related to their environment. We once had those creature powers, too, skill sets acquired when we still lived connected to those rich biomes and the creature life that existed within them. It was a time when we relied only on the sharply tuned acuity of our senses to make it through the events of each day or night. Eventually, as we grew more reliant on the fixtures of civilization and invested in their promising myths, we lost that finely honed store of knowledge that linked us to the web of natural life and our place within those systems.

So, where does that leave you and me?

Each of us must come to terms with the fact that we humans aren't what we used to be. We don't see, hear, or smell things as well as we used to. Or, for that matter, not as well as other animals do, either. We're more susceptible to viruses previously unknown. And we will likely have a much more difficult time coming to terms with the radical changes in climate, the freak weather, and the pandemics that the conflation of these events are bound to spawn. Scientists have no idea why humans seem to be on this declining evolutionary trajectory.* It may also have something to do with our inability to successfully cope with a climate of dwindling resources — conditions we've helped to produce — and that are

---

* Personal correspondence with Kevin Padian, Professor of Integrative Biology at the University of California, Berkeley, Curator of Paleontology, University of California Museum of Paleontology, former President of the National Center for Science Education from 2007 to 2008.

affecting our lives on a broad scale. Nevertheless, when compared to our distant relatives, we've lost some seemingly important advantages. We've become punier. Our arm and leg muscles aren't nearly as strong, pound for pound, as those of our ape relatives. Don't agree? Try wrestling with a full-grown chimp half your weight and size.

Spoiler alert: Bet on the ape.*

When comparing our hearing acuity to other animals, we can't come close when it comes to detecting certain high and low sounds. Bats and some toothed whale species echolocate using high frequencies we can't even begin to hear. They do this by sending out loud, short bursts of precisely targeted sound in ranges where the return echoes provide an acoustic snapshot of the target prey. The return signal instantly reveals all the information bats need in order to decide whether the targets are worth expending the energy to pursue. (Think of submarines and their range-finding sonar that was inspired by these critters.) Then there's the greater

---

* Personal correspondence with Kevin Padian.

wax moth, which can hear frequencies as high as 300kHz. For you musicians reading this, that's about six and a half octaves higher than the highest note on a piano and about four times higher than a young child with the full human range of hearing can detect. The ability of these animals to accurately target and process the information they receive gives new meaning to the term awesome.

In one lab test done in the late 1960s, while I was interning with the late marine scientist Dr. Thomas Poulter, a harbor seal in an indoor lab pool was able to perceive the difference between two coins the size of a quarter—one made of aluminum, the other of steel—using echolocation from twenty-five yards away! Underwater! Unless their habitat was free from human-induced noise, these marine mammals would have a hard time communicating in their natural environment. Where masking noise is introduced by boat propellers along with physically damaging ranging signals from high-tech military vessels, the echolocation precision of many marine mammal species suffers as does their ability to vocalize over normal ranges.

Elephants and some large whales (again) send out very low frequency vocalizations to communicate over long distances. When conditions are right, an elephant's low-frequency signals can travel through the air a couple of miles in a forest if unimpeded by human industrial sound like chain saws, generators, drilling and mining equipment, and large logging trucks. With the elephants' ground signals, the surface layer across the terrain vibrates as the signals are transmitted and received through the large pads of their feet. Moreover, under optimum conditions low-frequency elephant vocalizations could be detected up to twenty miles away (the distance across the widest part of Long Island)! Meanwhile, some whales' low-frequency voices are powerful enough to circle the globe if not blocked by landmass or human noise pollution in their marine biomes. Those particular whale voices are so low that we can't actually hear them. But we can *feel* the sounds viscerally if we're within range and in the water at the same time those signals are being transmitted.

Still, we humans retain the same hearing equipment that all other mammals have—the eardrum, the tiny middle ear bones we call the hammer, anvil, and stirrup, and the network of sensitive hair cells and nerves in the inner ear that sends those signals to the brain where they are sorted and given meaning or filtered out as being of little or no value (noise). With the presence of noise, our brains expend a lot of energy evaluating many useless signals that, nonetheless, have an effect on us, whether we want them to or not. We'll deal with those conditions later.

Even equipped with the same general listening tools as other mammals, our devolution to substandard hearing may be primarily due to our lopsided reliance on vision to engage with our surroundings. Or maybe it's just disuse. In the wild, acute hearing is crucial for detecting potential prey, the approach of predators, and other dangers. Not only did we use our hearing when we hunted, but—here's the kicker—it also served as an aural GPS to guide us through unfamiliar terrain at night without the aid of artificial light and where there was no way to navigate by starlight because of the dense forest canopy overhead. Think of that concept as a biophonic map. Aside from our ears, over time, we lost many of our best features—big muscles, extremely sharp eyes, and the ability to smell—all in a tradeoff for a large brain.

Natural environments aren't necessarily less complex than noisy urban habitats, although, if a wild biome is healthy, it's likely to be way more acoustically organized into neat sonic niches, with each critter or species' voice establishing its own special bandwidth or acoustic turf just like instrumental voices are organized in a musical composition. Think of the soundscapes of a particular place as a 24/7 environmental news report. It's where each habitat produces its own cohesive biophonic expression, an understandable narrative portrayed in an ancient protolanguage. Urban soundscapes, on the other hand, tend to be far more disorganized and incoherent.

Complexity is a key feature of urban anthropophonies. Walk through any construction zone in New York City where wrecking balls are taking down a building, water hoses are wetting down the dust clouds created by the collapsing walls, and compressors can be found running off roaring generators. Trucks, meanwhile, jockey in and out of the area removing debris. All this stuff is hopelessly loud with lots of competing and irritating sound sources. But, other than the incredible power of transformative human tools designed to improve on nature, and other than your body's aversive reaction to the din, other than signals of danger there is no clear message to be heard within all that racket. Even if we tried, our brains become overwhelmed when attempting to make sense of the chaos.

Natural and anthropogenic types of complexity differ between the two habitats making them fairly easy to distinguish from each other. Natural environments tend to be more organically (naturally) structured—an expressive refrain containing lots of detailed information, voices that have evolved to stay out of one another's acoustic turf. The other is human generated, utterly random, and assertively driven. One is healthful for you. The other, no matter how resilient you think you are, can literally make you ill.

In order to illustrate that point, I've created two spectrograms generated from the sound examples that follow this paragraph. I use spectrograms to help us visualize what we're hearing. These graphic illustrations of sound show you how each soundscape is constructed. In both examples the horizontal axis from left to right follows the soundscape through time; each example is less than twenty-five seconds in length. The vertical scale from the bottom to the top of the image, found on the right side, represents the frequency range of each voice, from low to high, with the entire range covering the full human frequency spectrum—20Hz (lowest) to 20kHz (highest). In the first one, from a once-healthy African habitat in Zimbabwe, you can actually *see* how sounds are elegantly arranged horizontally across the page from left to right, each within its own niche, and with contributions from many different animal sources as they generate a collective natural soundscape cohort, the biophony. Look at how well each vocally represented line establishes its own acoustic bandwidth distinguishing itself from others—just like that orchestral score mentioned earlier. The spectrogram doesn't tell you how loud each voice is, but it does emphasize the range of frequencies, differentiates the sources that create the sounds, and displays the relative times that those vocalizations occur in relationship to one another. In other words, you can now see and hear sound together as a continuous structure for the first time. Where the expression is graphically well partitioned, the habitat and resulting soundscapes tend to be healthy to be around. Now, look for the same kind of partitioning on the second spectrogram set, a typical construction zone that makes up part of a cityscape. Notice how all the competing sound sources mesh together without establishing any particular acoustic niches and with no available frequency territory or time slot left for a single living organism to vocalize. In this kind of chaos, there's no room for your voice to be heard, either. Where you hear or see those conditions, pay some attention. They are not beneficial environments in which to linger.

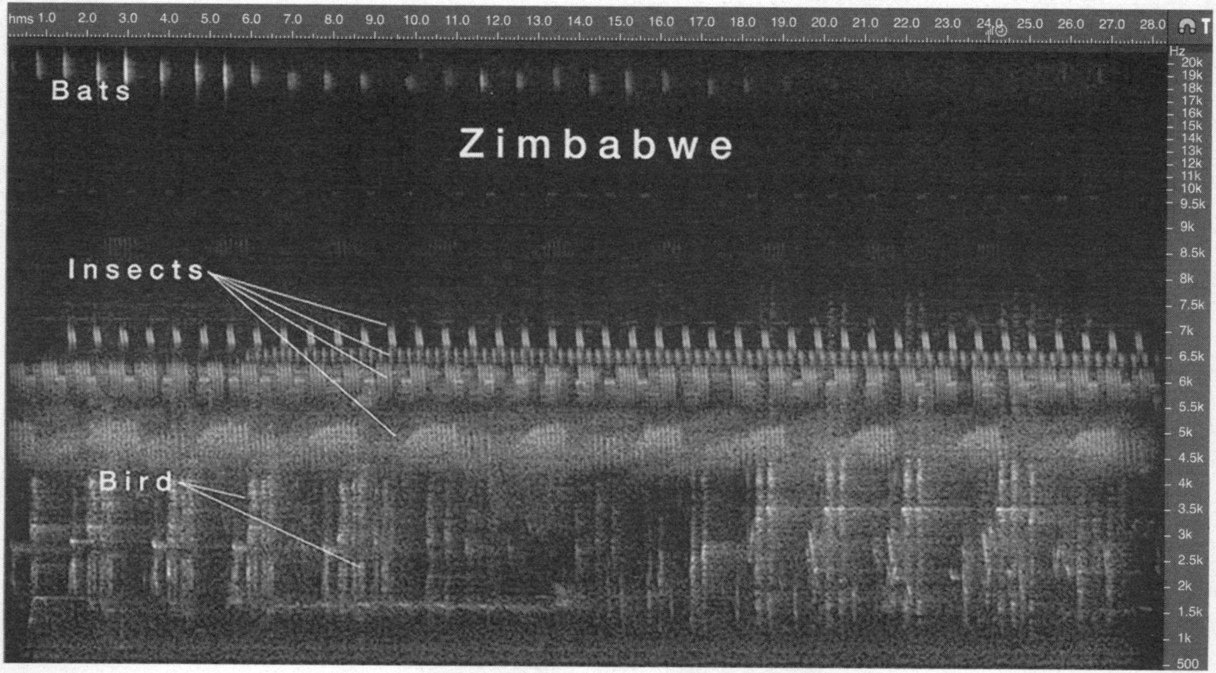
Zimbabwe
Bats
Insects
Bird
hms 1.0 2.0 3.0 4.0 5.0 6.0 7.0 8.0 9.0 10.0 11.0 12.0 13.0 14.0 15.0 16.0 17.0 18.0 19.0 20.0 21.0 22.0 23.0 24.0 25.0 26.0 27.0 28.0
Hz 20k 19k 18k 17k 16k 15k 14k 13k 12k 11k 10k 9.5k 9k 8.5k 8k 7.5k 7k 6.5k 6k 5.5k 5k 4.5k 4k 3.5k 3k 2.5k 2k 1.5k 1k 500

New York City
Construction

These patterns are clearly present in the visual examples of each acoustic expression. Ever wonder if there's any relationship between the ways we feel and act and the acoustic environments in which we choose to live and work? Noise-level readings from our phones would instantly prove that a Hell's Kitchen soundscape in New York City is certainly noisier than a particular wildlife area in south-central Zimbabwe at a location called Mungwezi Ranch, where the first example I just illustrated comes from. Both environments are sonically complex. You don't have to go to Africa to find examples of tranquil places: Breakneck Ridge, an hour north of Manhattan by train along the Hudson River, is possibly one such place, if you get there at the right time of day or night. Or try the Cape Cod National Seashore area in winter. Or the Adirondacks, a terrific wild area just to the west of Lake George and Lake Champlain, filled with wonderful natural habitats. You'll find quiet biomes in northern Wisconsin, Michigan, and the lake country of Minnesota, Algonquin Provincial Park in Ontario, the Canadian Maritimes, and remote sites in some of the US and Canadian national parks located throughout the North American west. Dive into our ancient pre-contact history and you'll find that our Native American and First Nations predecessors grew up immersed in the kind of soundscapes more like the one I've just described—multifaceted, inspiring, and consonant.

Although we who live in "civilized" environments eventually convince ourselves that we can tolerate the complexity of high levels of human-generated industrial noise, if we pause for a moment and think about it, the impressions that these chaotic environments leave behind are often intensely nerve-wracking. In contrast, natural habitats tend to be deeply enriching.

Random urban noise is not the only problem. Some types of noise are specifically focused and calculated to cause harm. Recently, for example, acoustic technology has been introduced that purposely uses noise to control your behavior. In the mid-1990s a Southern California company created a sound transmission device that could focus signals in a narrow beam, equivalent in broad concept to the way lasers focus light. At first, it was touted to be a solution to acoustic issues in large public spaces, like museums, where sound beams could be aimed narrowly, but without the signal "spilling" everywhere else in the building. Three problems: One, the sound quality was inferior. Two, in places with hard surfaces such as marble or concrete floors, the sound bounced around like billiard balls careening off the side cushions on a pool table. And, finally, the folks testing the device noticed that the transmitter itself sometimes made people feel dizzy or nauseated. Since the company had a difficult time selling the technology to their originally targeted general market, the sales group turned instead to the military and law enforcement and devised a way to reverse-spin plowshares into swords creating another application. They renamed it the LRAD (long-range acoustic device), an actual weapon touted as being noninvasive and momentarily uncomfortable but otherwise deemed to be safe.* Of course, given the way this device was employed as a tactical crowd-control tool, the claim of being noninjurious turned out to be unsupportable.

Originally designed for long-range communications at sea, where ships could securely and directly converse over distances of up to two miles (depending

---

* thedailybeast.com/how-the-lrad-went-from-a-pirate-deterrent-to-a -police-crowd-control-tool and defense-aerospace.com/article-view /feature/35072/pentagon-deploys-secret-sonic-weapon-in-iraq.html.

on which company literature you read) without their transmissions being intercepted, the company management calculated that they could enjoy broader acceptance and more lucrative government contracts if they promoted their device to the burgeoning military or paramilitary market. When the LRAD proved to have mixed results deterring pirates from attacking large tankers in the seas off East Africa, and the naval market proved to be too limited, they explored other applications. With small modifications, the company soon realized that one of the most efficient uses of the LRAD was in the manipulation of large gatherings of people. So, they marketed it to law enforcement as a new kind of sonic crowd-control weapon, one that has been used with some regularity even against our own population. During Pittsburgh's G20 protests in September 2009, for example, the LRAD was deployed to disperse crowds by exposing them to an extreme volume of directional sound. Its use led to legal action against the city, with one claimant receiving damages of $72,000 after suffering permanent hearing loss from contact with the signal. Other victims reported side effects from the short bursts of sound that included, among added medical issues, dizziness and nausea, loss of balance, and severe headaches.* There have been anecdotal reports of brain and internal organ damage as well. During the 2020 Black Lives Matter protests that occurred throughout the US, military-grade LRAD was also leveled at crowds to harmful effect.[†] With this application, the noise the device produces is calculated to incur a strong physical reaction: to disorient you, make you sick, and want to get out of the beam. The outcome results from the extremely distorted audio signal that LRADs transmit. If you're on the receiving end, no conditions are ideal. It's the harshest signal you're likely to hear. The damage to your ears if you choose to remain within range of the beam—unlike that of pepper spray to your eyes—may be permanent.

Here's another example that some of us encounter: Have you ever thought much about what disturbs you when you're trying to concentrate on a task you need to complete and there's acoustic distraction in your environment? Most people don't. Even those

---

* https://jolt.richmond.edu/2019/11/30/lrad-the-sound-of-possible-excessive-force.

† orlandosentinel.com/news/breaking-news/os-ne-orlando-george-floyd-protests-lrad-opd-20200625-vke7xwiggbg23llwetr4eggsz4-story.html.

of us who can multitask think that we can endure and successfully complete our undertakings even though the sound environment is not supportive. At this point, it's time to consider a typical soundscape scenario you might encounter.

Okay. You've got a paper to write for school, or a presentation to prepare for work tomorrow. You need to sort out your arguments, identify experts to back up your convictions, check credible websites for additional support, write compelling material that will pique the interest of your mentors, peers, or colleagues in the first few minutes and earn you well-deserved kudos when you finish. You settle in with your laptop and start writing. The moment you get a great idea and begin to flesh it out, a next-door neighbor's dog starts barking. You close the windows but it doesn't block out the yapping. Fifteen minutes go by, thirty. You're distracted and lose your train of thought. You move to another room, thinking it's far enough away from the incessant noise. Although the constant woofs are not terribly loud, the noise is as irritating as it is intrusive, and now you're just plain pissed. At this point, what are your choices?

If noise is an issue for you as it often is for me, one

of the conditions to consider when you're thinking of a place to work or live is how disruptive those signals can be. If you have the choice, take the time and patience to visit the potential work- or home site at all times of day and night to evaluate what the noise dynamics are and if they fit your lifestyle. These considerations include noise from neighbors, noise from the street, and even noise from the appliances in your apartment or house, such as vacuum cleaners, refrigerators, washers and dryers, radios and TVs, microwave ovens, hair dryers, and phones.

Again, it's not always loudness that makes for an irritating signal. Almost equally important is the *type* or *quality* of the sound when determining whether it's a useful signal. However, for the moment, let's give some attention to the sound levels in your environment. To get a handle on the volume of sound in your surroundings, enter "app for measuring ambient decibel levels" on your smartphone. You'll find a variety of helpful tools. Download one that suits you, and you'll get an immediate sense of how this plays out in your everyday environments. You'll be amazed. (I know this is a contradiction given that I've warned us to cool it with the phones, but bear with me.)

Look up "harmful noise levels" and you'll get something like:

Noise	Average Decibels (dB)
Normal room noise late at night	30
Night room noise with window cracked open	40
Normal conversation, background music	60
Office	70
Vacuum cleaner, average radio	75
Heavy traffic, window a/c, power lawn mower	80–89

(Note: noise above 85 is considered harmful)

Noise	Average Decibels (dB)
Subway, shouted conversation	90–95
Boom box, ATV, modified (straight-piped, no muffler) motorcycle	100–120
School dance	100–115
Chain saw, leaf blower, snowmobile	106–115
Symphony (loudest point)	70–117
Restaurants	85–120
Sports crowd, rock concert	120–130
Stock car races	130
Gunshot (.357 magnum thirty feet from your ears)	165

Getting back to noise levels in our everyday lives, let's dish about restaurants; an experience with sound common to most of us. In normal times, some establishments generate noise levels that are reasonable, averaging around 75–80dB. Others, like some newer venues, have sustained levels that approach 120dB, nearly eight times greater than what is normally comfortable. For comparison, that's within 10dB of a 747 jet at full throttle take-off power when the listener is standing thirty yards away!

Restaurant owners get that noise draws us to their establishments. Noise implies action to many people. We're drawn to it the same way your dog is attracted to a plate of kibble that she can't see but knows by scent is located on the kitchen floor of the apartment two floors below. Restaurateurs also get that the noisier their environment, the quicker the turnover. It's an obvious way of rushing you out the door while the maître d' and waitstaff are still pretending to be pleasant. It's Economics 101: gastro-capitalism. Think about it: The tables are close together, packing people into puny interior dining areas. No thought to social distancing in these joints. The interiors feature hard wall and floor surfaces certain to amplify the noise of the booming and competitive music. Diners scream at each other to be heard above the chaos and you'll have a hard time hearing your tablemates or the server as she tries to communicate the specials of the day. Alcohol service drives the levels even higher. According to Oxford University professor Charles Spence's research in the scientific journal *Flavour,* the food may be good, but you'll never be able to enjoy the flavors with the noise so distracting. Spence adds that noise actually alters your ability to taste. Some local publications, such as the *San Francisco Chronicle,* print noise level ratings as part of their restaurant reviews: one bell (intimate), two bells, three bells, four bells, cherry bomb (car-bleed). When Kat and I first walk into an establishment, I check our smartphone sound apps like dB Meter or Decibel X. If the level of the ambience exceeds 75dB, we're out of there. We use our devices mostly as a tool for comfort, not for the added and disrupting noise of social media.

Your sound level metering apps will come in handy no matter when or where you travel. It's obvious: The more tolerable and soothing the levels and types of signal, the less tired and stressed you'll feel, the more alert you will be to what's happening around you, and the better able you'll be to decide what to allow into your acoustic environment. If we were wearing earbuds to block unwanted noise, the potentially dangerous information Kat and I need to know about our surroundings might get lost. We know that by using them in that way, we might become targets for events we might not want to face, especially the types of random encounters that strike without warning in these unpredictable times. That kind of isolation is the last thing any of us needs.

If the ambient noise is really piercing, neither of us fight it. We just leave the area. Otherwise, we're gambling with headaches and anxiety, and potentially other risks as well. When your environment becomes shrill and chaotic, it's usually a consequence of many sources vying randomly for attention at the same time—some situations with potential for unpredictable outcomes. While what we think we see may be deceptive, our ears tell us the *truth* about when we're vulnerable. Keep them healthy and clear so that they'll be there when you need them. Get to know the signals. Take out the earbuds, put the phone away, do some ear-cleaning exercises by doing sound walks and distinguishing between all of the sound sources you experience, and keep your ears free of unnecessary distraction. Podcasts, Facebook, Instagram, Twitter, and texts can wait. The last thing your friends and contacts need is another badly lit photo of the latest Buddha bowl you've just ordered. What we do need to know is what's happening within range of what we can normally hear at any given moment. Social connection, communication, a sense of place are all enhanced by becoming consciously aware of your environment. Missing those details can eventually become a problem. Listen!

What are the most uncomfortable sounds in your environment?

Was it intentionally produced? It may have been unintentional, but would it be controllable if those creating the disturbance were made aware of the effect? Was it disturbing to you, individually, or is this a larger problem where a sizeable populated area that citizens live and work in is affected? What's the nature of those signals (i.e., how would you describe them)? If the irritant persists, what can be done to eliminate the problem?

CHAPTER 3

The Amazing Noise-Reduction Diet

Sound is a bit like food. Feed your body and soul the right nutrients, and you'll feel energized, amazed how that will transform and enhance your sense of well-being and consonance.

To get a better handle on what constitutes the right acoustic nourishment, let's begin with a two-part historical question: What might our remote ancestors have heard in their ancient homelands? And why do we need to know this? Aside from their own voices, our initial encounters were linked more deeply to natural-world influences. The first of these included non-biological natural sounds that I mentioned earlier, the geophony. The second consisted of biological voices, or biophonies. At the end of the last Ice Age, sixteen millennia ago, it would never have occurred to us that we were separate from our surroundings. Nor did we feel the need to compete with the soundscapes that defined our habitats. We blended in and became part of the acoustic fabric, meshing with our surroundings by imitating the sounds that individual creatures produced, learning from the choruses of organisms where our voices fit into the bio-spectrum, learning how to arrange sound, expressing rhythm by watching primates marking time on the buttresses of ficus (fig) trees, and imitating the actions of animals as they inspired us to move our bodies in sync. The sounds we responded to and reproduced early on were based on those that were biophonic. Thus, we learned to sing, dance, divide time, and to organize sound into early forms of musical expression as mimics. The connection also served as a palliative. Where can we find those restorative biomes now?

Bioregions like those of our ancestors are becoming scarce. Nevertheless, wholesome natural habitats can still be found. This is important, because if the soundscape is healthy, in support of the biosphere that surrounds it, it's likely to be relatively healthy for us human animals, too. When a disturbance occurs, such as the presence of a foreign critter or a predatory intruder, the whole biophonic expression of the habitat will change, alerting other organisms to heighten their awareness. At times the habitat will become eerily quiet as a defensive posture. Several species of birds or frogs will stop vocalizing, leaving just a few organic sounds. Ken Balcomb, founder of the Center for Whale Research in the San Juan Islands of Washington State, has observed that the masking of some loud-ranging signals from military vessels at sea and propeller cavitation from private boats cause killer whales and dolphins to lose their ability to communicate with other pod members and to find food through echolocation. The effect of this marine noise issue is thought to be a contributing factor to starvation in some pods.* Loud or abrasive noise has a similar disorienting effect when it prevents us from hearing the signals necessary for our survival.

Whether marine or terrestrial, the biophony expressed in those habitats may, in fact, express the precise nature of the disturbance. Animals in healthy habitats have evolved partitioned vocal

---

* https://projects.seattletimes.com/2019/hostile-waters-orcas-noise/.

ranges. As a result, their voices tend not to interfere with one another, thus carving out for themselves unique acoustic bandwidth they alone occupy. You know you're in a wholesome environment when discrimination among species is clearly audible on the one hand, and confirmed by spectrogram imaging on the other. With some exceptions, insects tend to settle on ranges in the upper frequencies or they vocalize at times when bandwidth is clear of other organisms' voices. Birds will tend to find acoustic turf mid-range, amphibians in the low–mid ranges, and large mammals, except some smaller whale species and manatees, generally vocalize in lower-ranging bandwidth. I describe this healthy acoustic structure because if you can locate habitats near you where these soundscapes exist, go there and listen. You'll come away actually feeling energized.

We don't have to disappear into the wild to find this type of sonic gift. Some of us may be lucky enough to live in a fairly quiet environment where we rarely hear sounds from highways, planes flying overhead, or our neighbors. On the other hand, urban locations, more common and replete with the usual background of cars passing on the streets nearby, kids playing outside and the requisite neighborhood canines, are the soundscapes many of us encounter in the biomes we inhabit. Cities are vibrant, ever-changing environments. Yet, even within those habitats we can find and enjoy quietude. Put on a pair of decent headphones and a program of natural soundscapes that you like, and you'll experience the healthful resonance of any number of wild habitats. There are lots of choices. The springtime sounds of deserts, lowland forested settings both temperate and tropical, the soundscapes of a summer evening, a seasonal stream, a mountain biome, even a recording of an urban dawn chorus.

If you're still craving noise, you won't have to go very far to contend with construction: someone down the street is using a circular saw, while another team of laborers is clearing a lot of debris with front-loaders, the equipment beeping each time it backs up with a load of dirt. Another crew is drilling and hammering bolts into a shear wall. This unintentional mixture of sound is not predictable. It's noisy. Unfortunately, the anthropophony begins at 6:30 A.M., at least an hour before it's supposed to. Nobody complains anymore. We think we've become accustomed to the din. We haven't. It's important for you to find a way to distance yourself from these signals. Lose sleep because of noise, and in a short period of time you won't feel terribly well.

When we hear these unstructured urban soundscapes, our mind reacts because the signals clash with our brain's need for order. Those that we receive contain combinations that we don't necessarily comprehend. We may generally recognize the source, but since the sounds themselves are not structured for focused messaging, our brains expend energy trying to filter and make sense of the signal. Incoherent electromechanical signals are not part of the natural environments from which we've evolved, so we fail. Consequently, when in the presence of acoustic incoherence we're often left feeling tired or stressed in response with no clear means to alter the effect. No matter how hard your brain tries to sort out the signals, a steady diet of urban noise is not easy to manage.

You may not be entirely conscious of the physiological impact on your system during these eruptions of noise. But it's likely that your blood pressure and glucocorticoid enzyme (stress indicator) levels will become measurably elevated. In this case, it happens when we find ourselves afflicted by disruptive types of soundscapes. We hear the noise, but the signals, other than affecting our physical well-being and coming across as annoying, produce no other obvious outcomes—in the beginning, at least. Other than affecting our sleep cycles, a garbage truck picking up trash at 4:30 in the morning outside your bedroom window means little or nothing to our mammalian brains.

Noise takes up space in the parietal and temporal lobes of our brain's processing centers. If its presence is too overwhelming and prolonged, you may well feel the anxiety that that noise induces and discover too late that it can weaken your immune system. These types of sound are not therapeutic.

Sometimes, even music that you'd think would be soothing and healing has the opposite effect because it is the wrong tempo, or the sound delivery system is distorted, or it is comprised of unfamiliar instrumentation. If it's performed in an uncomfortable setting it may add to a negative impact causing stress levels and heart rate to increase. The listener may simply despise the artist and his or her performance. And, finally, there's cultural bias: Where a performance of Beethoven's C# minor String Quartet would be engaging and reassuring for some, it might make a tween who loves Mamamoo or Blackpink

K-Pop nuts. Conversely, rapper Roddy Ricch's performance of "The Box" would seriously upset my Aunt Ida while others would be wholly riveted, because it delivers precisely the right acoustic momentum.

How do we deal with these contradictions? Eventually, what you like will help you decide how to control your sound environment, protect your ears, and keep you feeling more calm, relaxed, and focused. I'll explain how to choose healthy acoustic biomes more wisely in the next chapters. But first, we have to decide what kinds of sound environments we want to inhabit.

Just for the fun of it...

1. Pay careful attention to the ways you communicate within a field of noise.
2. How much energy do you expend...
   a. by talking louder?
   b. by being still trying to make out what another person is communicating?
   c. by waiting for the noise to diminish or go away, altogether?
   d. by getting exhausted and just abandoning the noise field altogether?

CHAPTER 4

Sound at the Edge
of the Forest

Ever give much thought to what types of sounds make you feel good? Maybe you have, but not in a fully conscious way. When that question is asked, most of us default to a choice of some type of music. But there's more to that question than meets the ear. For example: When most of us plan a vacation, one of the first considerations is to get to a place where you can unwind and relax—far away from the noisy environments of our everyday lives. Could be a place by the ocean or a lake in the mountains. Or it could be a remote spot in the desert, or a cabin in the woods. These ideals really exist. But then we complicate our plans filling our precious downtime with activities. I'm astonished by the number of people I've met who haven't even tried to imagine spending free moments without having to organize something to do. To be fair, the subject of true respite is not high on our cultural, emotional, or physical fitness priority lists. People will readily flock to yoga and Pilates classes, but how many show up for soundscape therapy or take a sound-walk? From the anecdotal interviews I've conducted, most folks, young and old, seem vaguely curious about quietude or finding an escape from noisiness. It's just not at a level to pursue beyond a passing curiosity. So, let's cut to the chase and identify some of the most nourishing types of soundscapes that would sustain you and that you will want to check out.

For a lot of us, these choices are very personal. One size does not fit all. However, there are some soundscape environments that appear to be more beneficial than others. You may want to try some by yourself. These hints come from sources that we don't normally think of or read about. What is surprising is that these groups have been using these soundscapes as antidotes for thousands of years. There are other examples, but let's imagine what these places might conjure for you.

Members of the Ba'Aka tribe, a group of

forest-dwelling Pygmies who live in the most remote section of the Dzanga-Sangha rain forest located in western Central African Republic (CAR), best convey this idea because it is such a deeply embedded feature of their lives. The rain forest biome has long been home to this seminomadic ensemble that traditionally relied solely on the resources the habitat provided to them, the bush meat they hunted for food and the wild plants they harvested for additional sustenance and medicines. The forest was there to supply whatever they needed although Ba'Aka lived relatively light on the land.

One morning in 1984 in New Jersey, an American musicologist named Louis Sarno happened to be listening to a radio program of Ba'Aka music. He was so captivated by the beauty of the music that he sold everything he owned, bought a one-way ticket to Bangui (the capital of the CAR), a recorder and some microphones, and cut most ties with his birthplace, friends, and family. Once on the ground in his newly adapted country, Sarno traveled for several days until he finally caught up with the tribe all but hidden in their rain forest home.

Of the many remarkable attributes of Sarno's life as a musical anthropologist and field recordist, one in particular made me think long and hard about the connection between the biophonies of the natural world and their restorative properties. In fact, my own experience was only amplified by Louis's narrative.

As Sarno told the story, during the late decades of the twentieth century a second wave of colonialism, including large conglomerates from Asia and the EU, began large-scale resource removal from the Ba'Akas' home territory. With accelerated logging of hardwood forests, extraction of diamonds, oil, and poaching of ivory from the elephant families of the surrounding jungle, the cash economies imposed on the country's ancient cultures by major companies replaced the small-scale as-needed traditional barter exchanges more familiar to the groups like the Ba'Aka. Drawn into the competitive economic and resource-driven models of the West and Asia, tribal members now had to purchase their meager necessities within the imposed cash systems in order to thrive. To acquire enough hard currency, males were enticed into the forest to illegally hunt bushmeat protein for the miners, loggers, and the administrative personnel, and elephant ivory for export to the black markets of the US and Asia. Meanwhile, the women were lured into prostitution. The neo-capitalistic trade-offs and intimate contact with the foreigners shredded the fragile social and economic structure of their community and introduced levels of trauma and disease not previously known. The strain on Ba'Aka culture caused many members to become quite ill or to die, raising the question of how they could mitigate the physical and emotional crises that now confronted them.

To manage this dilemma, Ba'Aka did what they had always done when faced with turmoil and illness. They disappeared all at once deep into the forest—sometimes for months on end—in an effort to separate themselves from the colonial noise and to heal in secret locations where their forest was still intact. The shamans, who had retained the ancient knowledge of which herbs and vegetation affected certain diseases and mental conditions, were still able to ply their magical art and craft. And, most important, they still understood how to integrate the biophonies and geophonies of the forest as curatives for just about everything else. With the biophonies serving as a natural karaoke orchestra with which they performed, the Ba'Aka would reinstate their ritual songs and dances, again finding solace in the reanimated spirits that could be found everywhere. After sufficient quiet and healing time, the tribal members would reemerge from the forest, healthy and vibrant, only to engage once again with the downward spiral of civilized contact.

During the nearly thirty-five years Sarno and I worked together, what struck me most of all was the way in which the Ba'Aka, dependent on their ancient connection to the rain forest, were able to sever their addictive ties to civilization and restore some measure of sanity back into their lives, if only momentarily. Can you imagine a healing sonic environment for yourself? What would that sound like?

I grew up in a large midwestern industrialized city in the mid-twentieth century, during a war-time economy, a time when it produced enormous amounts of military and, later, consumer goods. As a kid, while I knew a lot about mechanical things, I hardly knew what a forest was or anything much about the animal world. The only exceptions were the mental images I got from fairy tales my dad read to me when I was very little. Aside from occasional summer trips to a beach, a few weeks in camp when I was very young, or a quick tour of a national park, my family's draw to the wonders of the natural world was not a priority.

Born with a chronic ADHD condition that has tracked well into adulthood, I was desperate to find ways to feel less anxious and depressed, having been dismissed as less worthwhile than my peers. I was a mediocre student because the disorder left me dyslexic and incapable of concentrating, issues I still confront today. I'm certain that I disappointed my parents, never quite able to meet either their unspoken or stated expectations. And they, in response, weren't shy about calling out my deficiencies, which didn't instill a lot of self-confidence. At times, there seemed to be no exit, no way out, until that moment in a Northern California forest when I first experienced the power of a forest biophony and felt such an overwhelming sense of relief both physically and emotionally. It was a safe remedy I would rely on for the rest of my life. Later visits to wild habitats near and far helped validate that first experience, one where a sense of anxiety that had so totally dominated my life was now manageable. No medication, prescribed or otherwise, came close to that woodland therapy.

My asthma, affected by tree and grass pollen in

spring, and my allergy to cats and dogs, diminished to the point where I could tolerate these things in ways that otherwise would have landed me in an ICU just a few years before. I was so embarrassed to share this secret with others that I rarely spoke of the issue until very recently. While there were a few murmurs about natural soundscapes in the literature from folks like Thoreau, Paul Shepard, Mary Oliver, Aldo Leopold, Rachael Carson, and Ellen Glasgow, it never occurred to me that other people might have experienced the same kind of relief until I met Sarno and he told me stories about the Ba'Aka forest healing practices. I am not alone.

Much later, around the year 2000, I learned about *shinrin yoku,* Japanese forest bathing—a quest through time spent in forested habitats for more intimate and spiritual connections to the natural world. A simple nature therapy program introduced in the early 1980s by Yoshifumi Miyazaki, a university professor and the codirector of the Center of Environmental Sciences at the University of Chiba in Japan, is a largely passive methodology that I was already familiar with from my own encounters with wildlife in the field. *Shinrin yoku,* loosely translated, means "taking in the medicine of the forest." This evidence-based wellness practice was a direct response to declining health in the Japanese population at the time. The healing energies of the natural world have been known for millennia. This practice is another simple yet powerful way for us to tap into those healing energies that are readily available to all of us—particularly those related to the sonic properties of natural habitats. Extensive research shows that forest bathing can offer relief from anxiety and depression, bestow a deeper sense of mental relaxation, better sleep, and an increased feeling of gratitude for being alive, and deliver an overall sense of well-being. When forest bathing, we walk into designated areas after first being given a set of carefully crafted invitations, ways to slow down and to experience the more than human world through a variety of new techniques and our senses. You don't have to cover much distance, but you do need to find a forest. Miyazaki's writings and the stories of the Ba'Aka confirmed the efficacy of this practice, a process that had taken me many years to acquire. Most of all, it helped me give voice to my own experiences.

Shinrin yoku inspires us to make time for lei-surely strolls in tranquil wooded areas, the simple idea being that a break from the noise of our tech-nosphere in exchange for a closer relationship to natural-world phenomena conveys enormous benefits.*† It's a contemporary antidote to the distractions brought on by the constant acoustic dissonance emblematic of our presence.

Richard Louv, *Last Child in the Woods* author, reminds us of the consequences of denying our young children access to wild habitats. These are places where kids can connect with the elemental roots of their lives with a path to wholesome maturity within their respective cultures.‡

The use of forest soundscapes as an aural map was mentioned in the second chapter. But there's another example I'd like to share: Bruce Albert, the French anthropologist who has worked intimately with the Yanomami tribe, describes the forest soundscape as a narrative of a place, an ancient idea

---

* Yoshifumi Miyazaki, *Shinrin-yoku, the Japanese Art of Forest Bathing,* Timber Press, 2018.

† Caoimhe Twohig-Bennet and Alan Jones, "The Health Benefits of the Great Outdoors: A Systematic Review and Meta-analysis of Greenspace Exposure and Health Outcomes," *Environmental Research,* vol. 166, October 2018: 628–37.

‡ nytimes.com/2020/06/23/parenting/nature-health-benefits-corona virus-outdoors.html?

germane to all of us: "It is then essentially the use of hearing which allows them (Yanomami) to detect [the animals'] presence and their movements, in the undergrowth or the canopy of trees. It is therefore easy to understand that the acoustic knowledge of the forest environment of Amerindian hunters is considerable since their youngest age, but also that the concert of animal sounds which permanently encompasses them deeply permeates their language, their cosmology and their sense of well-being. The acoustic experience of the Yanomami Indians of northern Brazil, with whom I have had the privilege of interacting for several decades, offers a good example of this influence of the biophony of the tropical forest on the lived knowledge of the Amazonian peoples. I will mention a few examples here, from the dialogue of hunters with the voices of the forest to the myth of the origin of animal languages, including the learning of ceremonial and shamanic songs.

Along their hunting or gathering routes, the Yanomami maintain a constant dialogue with the multiplicity of voices from the forest. Their rapt attention to forest biophony is the object of constant awareness while they are always quick to express mimicry in response to their non-human interlocutors. This extreme acoustic concentration is, moreover, doubled by the permanent deciphering of an elaborate system of sound correspondences that they associate with the notion of *heã*. The hunters designate by this term the songs, cries and calls of very many birds (but also of amphibians and certain insects) which they consider as acoustic clues that can reveal the presence in the forest of prey, of fruits or plants associated with them. As one of them summed up laconically to me: *Urihiha yaro pë ã waroho hwai tëhë, yaro pë heã kua yama ki kuu,* "When many animal voices speak in the forest, we say they are the sound signals of game. In this system of sound correspondences the cooing of the fasciated batara reveals the presence of a tapir, and the rolled song of the black-tailed trogon announces a herd of collared peccaries. The approach of the spider monkeys is signaled by the shrill two tones of the small blue-headed parrots, the passage of a red dagger (deer) by the jerky trill of the smoky climber, while the hissing sound flute of the bambla troglodyte announces the proximity of a nine-banded armadillo. In the vegetal area, the melodious song of the cocoa blackbird..." and so on. "The complex network of associations between indicative animal voices and the presence of game or useful plants in the *heã* Yanomami forest thus constitutes an acoustic locating system taught from childhood which, both permanent and constantly moving, is always able to guide hunters and collectors within the 'large animal orchestra' of the forest area."*

In our relatively short time as members of the Anthropophonocene, we've largely sheltered within an expanding bubble of our own technological din, drawn to virulent destructive signals and dismissing those that may well be restorative. Especially problematic is exposure to loud sound signatures present since the advent of the Industrial Revolution, a fairly recent period when humans began to push urban density to extremes and coincidentally cranked the levels of sound to brandish our newfound sense of power. Now, however, we're seeing another effect of

---

* Excerpt from "The Polyglot Forest" by Bruce Albert, first published in the exhibition catalog *The Great Animal Orchestra,* Fondation Cartier pour l'art contemporain, Paris, 2016. Used with permission.

Extrait de "La Forêt Polyglotte" par Bruce Albert, publié pour la première fois dans le catalogue d'exposition Le Grand Orchestre des Animaux, *Fondation Cartier pour l'art contemporain, Paris, 2016.*

those human concentrations with the spread of the COVID-19 virus. In contrast, and with many of us off the streets, our urban centers suddenly became very quiet for a time. Is there something to be gained from those moments?

The examples I've just described—two from ancient cultures and the other from a contemporary one—provide a timeless summons into the recesses of the human psyche. No matter when or where we live, this reflection obliges a form of nurture obtainable only through direct links to and involvement in the operational embrace of the natural world. Take your pick. Either approach works. The natural world has many open portals.

For those in urban centers hearing for the first time the structure of natural sound with everything so quiet, imagine how you'd feel taking a break now and then and ambling off into a forest that was set aside for its relatively tranquil properties at all hours of the day, all seasons of the year.

Folks worldwide have begun to hear what's therapeutically possible within these soundscapes especially when the competition with high noise levels humans generate is diminished. For example, a park in Taipei is noted for being one of the most tranquil urban parks in the world. Located in Taiwan, an island of 22 million people, it is one of the world's most densely populated places. Yangmingshan National Park is located just north of the capital, Taipei, and is home to rare aquatic plants, expressive frogs, and the endemic Formosan blue magpies, among many other vocal organisms. This subtropical biome consists of more than forty square miles of mountainous terrain, as well as forests interspersed with hiking trails, and even features pristine hot springs. It's a place where nearby urban dwellers can go to bathe in soundscapes of elegant biophonies and where the human noise rarely exceeds a sound pressure level of 45dB, equivalent to background noise in a very quiet bedroom.*

The power of these natural voices is still amazing, to me, one who's been studying the effects for years. Young children, who have nothing acoustically in their early memory banks to compare, are remarkably shaped by the initial impact of these gentle sounds. That's because biophonies are possibly embedded in our DNA and the resonances

---

* cntraveler.com/story/taipei-is-home-to-the-worlds-first-urban-quiet -park?utm_source=onsite-share&utm_medium=email&utm_camp aign=onsite-share&utm_brand=conde-nast-traveler.

may elicit vague memories of our evolutionary past. The exchanges between wild animals and children enliven their encounters with the living world with a sense of wonder and delight.

In order to maintain that sense of miraculous presence—the one I alluded to in the introduction—you will not only need to scope out natural habitats that speak to your need for tranquility, but you'll also want to spend time engaging with them. If you have the wherewithal to record your experiences in the wild, treat yourself to the result with some measure of enjoyment when you play back the soundscapes you've collected. And you can do that within the confines of your own dwelling.

Consider healthful ways to engage acoustically

Identify a nearby habitat that's peaceful—ideally an environment relatively free of urban noise. Go there safely. Eliminate the distractions. Hang out. When physically traveling to that spot isn't possible, link a pair of earphones to your laptop or phone, close the door to your room, darken the space, and immerse yourself in one of the better-produced natural sound albums now available online. Pick a sound type that you imagine to be the most relaxing. Waves along the shore of a freshwater lake. Water in a stream. A tropical rainstorm. A dawn chorus in a temperate forest. A springtime evening chorus in the American Southwest. Either way, engaging with natural-world soundscapes will make a difference. That said, some types of music work, too. Keep in mind, as mentioned earlier, that because music is tagged with cultural bias, it may not be as effective as natural sound.

CHAPTER 5

Healing Comes in Waves

In the last chapter I compared the similarities between old and new therapies and the noises of civilization. This chapter is devoted to the actual spaces that help us feel more relaxed and comforted. After all, the effects we want to achieve are dependent on the choices we make. Primal or modern, there's no alternative to solo time in the woods. But for many of us it's not always possible to go.

Yet, we only have to turn back to the natural world for inspiration to create more beneficial acoustic spaces for ourselves. To begin with, if neighborhood noise is an issue, urban planners now suggest the planting of certain types of trees to help mitigate the problem. Yup, trees. The BBC science and environment programming department recently reported that planting larch trees, a type of conifer, tends to quiet things down in neighborhoods. It cuts reverberation and absorbs noise with its thick bark.* We've managed to address those conditions in interior spaces with design techniques that include sound-absorbent drywall and even new types of paint, not to mention different types of fabric.

The spaces that we humans typically inhabit, whether they're offices, homes, or hotel rooms, are not usually created to produce ideal noise reduction. Until recently, neither architects nor interior designers gave that issue much thought. Yet, if you value your health and well-being, you may want to listen carefully to the ambience in the vicinity of your work, living, and recreational spaces.

Next time you go to work, sit or stand quietly for a moment in your work space. Tune in to your surroundings. Is there any distracting or uncomfortable acoustic feature that stands out? Would moving to a different area or room help alleviate that problem? If allowed, would putting a small rug on the floor, or soft, absorbent material over the surfaces of your

---

* bbc.com/news/science-environment-52139333.

work space make a difference? When you become proactive about your sonic environment, you'll find that a more peaceful space will help you concentrate better. You can make a big difference in the quality of your work with just a few minor superficial changes. Claim your peaceful spaces.

After we lost our rural home and everything else in the October 2017 Northern California fires, we had to search for a temporary place to live. Kat and I came across many dwellings located on well-traveled streets. Some structures included windows made up of single-paned glass and doors that offered little protection from the intruding mechanical sounds outside. But there were other places, located in similar neighborhoods, insulated so that street noises were diminished. These latter environments seemed much more peaceful and soothing to us. Designed to be more tranquil, they were nearly always more inviting, beckoning for us to linger. By opting for those habitats, we could begin to control the sound in our living space, and the amount of noise we allowed simply by how much we chose to keep the windows open and our media delivery systems active.

Even if you live in an urban setting, with a bit of ingenuity and not much cost you can create a DIY intimate acoustic space that will leave you feeling both calmed and secure. Most important, make sure that your space is or can be made fairly non-reverberant by "tuning" it. Reverberation creates the illusion that sound is louder and bigger. At the same time important acoustic signals that you may need to hear become diffused and less distinct. Most habitable structures come with parallel walls, ceilings, and floors. Enhance those features with hard, reflective surfaces and the rooms will tend to be quite echoey with sound literally bouncing off the walls. So, you'll also want to break up the parallel façades with sound-absorbent fabric or other fabric-covered panels to alter the contours of the room. The more you do to tone down the reverberation, the more intimate your area will feel. Your ears will tell you when the room is sufficiently tuned—it'll be the moment you're comforted when hanging out within the space you've created. It will feel more tranquil.

After the 2017 fires, Kat and I moved to a small community of around eleven thousand people not far from Wild Sanctuary. There we found ourselves in the midst of a real-life neighborhood of closely situated small houses—our first city-like experience in almost thirty years. The place we finally rented initially posed some new problems, such as traffic and neighbors just doing their thing. To come to terms with those changing conditions, several mornings a week at first light in the spring, I'd go out for a long walk to clear my head and prepare for the daily noise debris field that lay ahead. Part of the delight of those moments was hearing the reassuring songs of urban birds as darkness graduated to dawn twilight and the soon-to-be visible sun. Mostly the animal orchestra consisted of common northern hemisphere urban critters: American robins, song sparrows, white- and orange-crowned sparrows, towhees, mockingbirds, and house finches in various combinations. If it was early enough, a pair of great horned owls would cover the lower mid-range and bass register, calling back and forth between themselves—the female's voice a bit higher in pitch than her mate's. These choruses always made for soothing companions as I walked the nearly empty streets and dirt paths of our neighborhood. In cities, it's the quietest time of day and a lovely period to be outside. Try it. Even if you're not a morning person, that act alone will make you feel refreshed and reconnected to the living world. You don't need the excuse of a pandemic to make that happen. Spend some valuable time each day in the peaceable quest of listening.

One of the key acoustic remedies I learned when creating sound installations for public spaces was to first address the problem of reverberation in the places we were transforming. The extent to which we were able to convince the exhibit designers to mitigate that issue alone determined the degree to which the installation was successful. By amending reverberation, these spaces were able to influence the behavior of large groups of young visitors because they were passively denied the reflection of their voices. As a result, the youngsters became much quieter and more reverent when visiting those modified environments. A non-reverberant space tends to reduce the desire to talk or play loudly. The same goes for those spaces in your home, a restaurant, or in a school classroom. I emphasize this factor as probably the most important element in an enriched interior space where acoustics plays a role.

You can be confident that when you are able to still the everyday exterior noise that clutters your mind, your interior weather will feel much less turbulent. Just remember that noise comes in all shapes, sizes, and from lots of sources. In the process of transforming those waves of acoustic energy, you will introduce practical solutions that personalize and make intimate the spaces you choose to inhabit. Then you'll be able to fill your mediated environment with sounds you like in ways that soothe rather than detract or irritate. All things being more or less acoustically balanced, the high blood pressure and sense of anxiety you sometimes feel should be greatly reduced just by that simple act.

From the list of distracting or irritating sounds you've noted while taking your sound walks, imagine the kinds of spaces that would free you from the impact of those annoyances merely by shutting them out. In our case, after the fire, one of the many rentals Kat and I found ourselves in was an oddly laid out space with fairly cramped rooms and hard, reflective wall and floor surfaces. The reverberation was disorienting, and we had to figure out ways to rectify that. Then I remembered the impressions of the room my parents decided was perfect for my first few years. The space also served as an ideal environment for penance, the quarters to which I was exiled when I misspoke or misbehaved. After a few banishments, I transformed it both in my imagination and reality into a nurturing refuge from all of the noise that otherwise diverted my attention. Although I certainly wasn't equipped to design a noise-free space, with the addition of just a few personal items strategically placed, I managed to convert it to one more intimate and welcoming. It became a safe haven with little or no interruption from the street, a place where I could practice violin, at once removed from the harsh arguments between my parents (my sister was too little to engage then), and the house's cacophony of clanging dishes, pots and pans, the thrum and whine of the old Bendix clothes washer in the basement, the Hammond organ "stings" of afternoon radio soap operas, flushing toilets, running faucets, the creaking of the wooden stairs as Mom or Dad ascended or descended them, and the clicks and squeaks that signified the opening and closing of doors.

When I began to study violin, I knew instinctively from the outset that my room was too "alive" because of the hard surfaces. By throwing blankets on the floor, or draping them over the bed and closing the curtains and blinds I made the acoustics more conducive to practicing because the sound of the instrument became more responsive. Realizing that I could control the sonic features of the room to some extent, that tiny shelter served as the model for all my favored spaces that would follow.

Jumping quickly ahead seventy-five years or so, in our first post-fire rental home, there was no real area for a tranquil listening room where I could work. For the makeshift sound studio I fashioned a space out of the smallest bedroom, a 110-square-foot area with just enough room for two speakers, a computer, and a small mixing desk. I brought in some used baffles and curtains to cover the walls and added a thick, sound-absorbent carpet made of remnants from a local carpet dealer. With just a few square feet left for me to sit, it worked. I could close the door, trigger a recording from Alaska and instantly transport myself back to some remote exotic spot reimagined through the strains of its biophony, an expansive illusion of wild spaces enhanced by the effects of wind, hundreds of bird species including a pair of Arctic loons and an Arctic fox, an illusion far more vivid than a two-dimensional photo. If the recordings were good enough, I could even conjure the scent of tundra tea that permeated our campsite as it brewed over the Coleman stove, an infusion that Kat and I drank faithfully each day at

4 P.M. In an instant, by adding a single particular soundscape, I was able to convert a small bedroom into a sonic illusion of wide Arctic expanses, or any other wild biome I chose from my archive. Natural soundscapes have those transformative powers. At the same time, I get that you might prefer a reassuring musical example. Again, either choice works.

But supposing you don't have that extra area? What then?

You don't need a room to do this. Decent Bluetooth headphones or earbuds will do if your playback system delivers respectable quality. Just keep the volume set at reasonable levels to protect your ears. The key here is to make the spaces you inhabit restorative by playing to your acoustic needs, whether they be the office space where you work, your home, or where you relax, play, or eat.

If you can, treat yourself to an extended unplugged meditative session. Choose a site where there is no smartphone or Wi-Fi, no TV, Spotify, or Pandora, nothing electromechanical. Break the internet and phone connection urge. If you're agile and game enough, and have the luxury of time, it could be a hike along the Appalachian Trail in the eastern US or part of the John Muir Trail in the Sierra Nevada Mountains, one that winds its way through Sequoia/Kings Canyon and Yosemite National Parks—more than two hundred miles in all. That walk in the woods, or forest bathing, makes a big difference. Birdsong, insects, or the drone of frog sound is quite magical to meditate to. Alternatively, you could simply shut off the noise sources in your home and settle in for a well-deserved respite where you live. Don't go for silence. Silence means no sound and it doesn't exist in any part of the natural world in which we evolved. Aim, instead, for tranquility, a term that British soundscape ecologist Chris Watson refers to meaning a condition often mistaken for silence, but instead, assumes an environment that is both calming and remedial.

Humans have been trying to describe soundscapes since we first gathered in large groups that ultimately grew into cities. It even shows up in poetry. In the United States, a contemporary city soundscape would be only partially familiar to Walt Whitman, who wrote eloquently of nineteenth-century urban anthropophonies in his classic poem "Song of Myself" more than 160 years ago:

Now I will do nothing but listen,
To accrue what I hear into this song, to let
    sounds contribute toward it.

I hear bravuras of birds, bustle of growing
    wheat, gossip of flames,
clack of sticks cooking my meals,
I hear the sound I love, the sound of the
    human voice,
I hear all sounds running together, combined,
    fused or following,
Sounds of the city and sounds out of the city,
    sounds of the day and night,
Talkative young ones to those that like them,
    the loud laugh of
work-people at their meals,
The angry base of disjointed friendship, the
    faint tones of the sick,
The judge with hands tight to the desk, his
    pallid lips pronouncing
a death-sentence,
The heave'e'yo of stevedores unlading ships by
    the wharves, the
refrain of the anchor-lifters,

The ring of alarm-bells, the cry of fire, the
    whirr of swift-streaking
engines and hose-carts with premonitory tin-
    kles and color'd lights,
The steam-whistle, the solid roll of the train
    of approaching cars,
The slow march play'd at the head of the asso-
    ciation marching two and two,
(They go to guard some corpse, the flag-tops
    are draped with black muslin.)

I hear the violoncello, ('tis the young man's
    heart's complaint,)
I hear the key'd cornet, it glides quickly in
    through my ears,
It shakes mad-sweet pangs through my belly
    and breast.

I hear the chorus, it is a grand opera,
Ah this indeed is music—this suits me.

I wonder what Whitman would make of the
soundscapes of modern American cities with police,
fire, and ambulance sirens, gunshots, helicopters,

commercial and private aircraft, construction, automobiles and alarm systems, lawn mowers, leaf blowers, and straight-piping vehicles, each one the sound mark of unrelenting commerce and a struggle for individual recognition? Yet, as changes brought about by the COVID-19 US shutdown confirmed, that organically beautiful fabric of natural sound competing for a place in the sonic structure still exists.

Eliminating noise results in positive effects. Before 9/11, Kat and I simply accepted the intrusions of jet and private aircraft, helicopters and distant road traffic in our valley as part of the normal sound signatures of our biome—a necessary outcome of the compulsively driven world and times we live in. But on September 12, 2001, the day after the Twin Towers were hit, the skies across the US were empty of most aircraft and very few cars or motorcycles were on the road. As we sat outside in our backyard, talking about the horrors we had witnessed on television, we also came to terms with how lucky we were to be safe with each other. At one point we came to a place in our conversation where there was nothing more to say. We remained quiet without speaking for a long time, completely drained, just listening to the day unfold. For the first time that late in the season, we remarked on the fragile but present daytime bird-saturated soundscape we'd never been aware of before at that time of year. With all the forces of commerce momentarily stilled, we were able to hear the remaining biophonic voice of our own habitat—bestowed on us as a kind of threnody. Which begs the question: How the hell did those birds know to sing just then? Or have they been crying out to us all along and we couldn't hear them through the strata of noise we can't seem to live without?

Many factors play a role in the ways biophonies are expressed in a given location: topography, weather, time of day or night, surrounding vegetation, total numbers of species and vocal sources, and season all help determine the many ways those signals play out. As a result of climate change, the content of these sites is beginning to shift more quickly and dramatically from place to place and year to year. Generally speaking, wild soundscapes are produced within boundaries we're not usually conscious of. One of these boundaries defines the total acoustic field from which you can detect sound coming from any direction. In other words, from a standing position in one location, what nondomestic organic sounds can you pick up from any source? Now, what human-generated sounds, no matter how far away, can you detect from that spot? Make a note of them on a piece of paper. In wild terrestrial habitats, these ranges make up the boundaries defined by acoustic turf. The combination of all those features delineates an acoustic border, whether the habitats within are classified as forests, deserts, high plains, mountains, tropical or temperate rain forests, and even marine biomes. The shapes of these borders will not likely be square, circular, or rectangular grids, the common geometric shapes humans tend to impose on an otherwise shape-shifting world. They're more likely to be amoeba-like and mutable over time. They expand and contract. One aspect of the biophonic narrative tells us that the natural world is not constrained to the limits of our organizational models. It generates margins all its own—ones we may never fully comprehend.

With wild habitats declining, transformed into parking lots, shopping malls, megawarehouses, and other signs of what some call progress, tiny bits of wildlife still survive to repopulate and adjust to the transformed patches left to them in urban and suburban areas. The persevering ones have no choice. Those, like us, that can adjust their vocal behavior to accommodate to altered environments may pay a price. In order to overcome the pandemonium we generate, all of these organisms struggle for purchase with some risk of discovery and danger, the result being that many tend to reconfigure their vocal patterns. Some become more quiet—rarely visible except on motion-sensing still or video cameras.

During the first six months of the COVID-19 pandemic in 2020, researchers observed a significant change in the vocalizations of urban birds. Since human activity in the biomes they studied had become much more calm from a human perspective, the birds didn't have to expend so much energy to be heard. Therefore, they could sing at a lower volume.* In more normal times, unless urban wildlife evolves to express itself with vocalizations that exceed in level or shift in timbre the anthropogenic noise around them, we won't hear them as often as we would in other, more naturally scaled environments, or unless our city anthropophonies become more muted. We, on the other hand, to preserve our sanity, must come to terms with the larger view of how these human-generated

---

* tpr.org/2020-09-24/scientists-find-the-quiet-of-pandemic-shutdowns-has-made-birds-change-their-tunes.

noise issues affect every one of us. Then we need to find the collective will to alter these negative trends. To a large extent, human health and the health of our wildlife habitats depend on those decisions.

As I was writing the other day, I received an email from a friend with a link to an article, the subject of which was the noisiest city on the planet. To illustrate the point, there was a picture of a wall of speakers that appears to be some ten to fifteen feet high and so wide that it failed to fit in the frame horizontally. Passing in front of the speaker wall are a couple of young fellows on a motorbike. The passenger riding on the backseat has his hands over his ears, presumably trying to reduce the oppressive levels that they couldn't otherwise avoid as they passed. This particular prize goes to Delhi, India, although the award is arguable and could go to any of several locations in Asia, Europe, Africa, or North America. But back to my main point: According to the article, the residents of Delhi suffer hearing loss equivalent to those typically nineteen years of age or older, who live in places where there are also very high levels of noise.*

---

* Matthew Keegan, "Where Is the World's Noisiest City?," *The Guardian,* March 8, 2018. The study was sponsored by the Rocke-

Shanghai, China, a city of nearly 25 million inhabitants, tends to be quieter because the authorities there have eliminated a major contributor to city noise in a dramatic and rather authoritarian way. Instead of combustion engine motorbikes, scooters, and cycles, the government has mandated that mechanically driven two-wheeled vehicles be electric powered. The immediate impression is that the street noise levels are much quieter, making Shanghai, crowded as it is, a far less stressful place to walk outside in many parts of the city — assuming the air is clear of the unremitting blanket of industrial smog that has plagued their atmosphere. Pedestrians merely have to pay attention when they try to cross the street. Scooter drivers assume they have the right of way, and you won't *hear* them coming if you're an otherwise distracted pedestrian. Compared to the incredible noise levels on the streets of Paris, one of the loudest cities in Europe, Shanghai is a sonic Shangri-La.

One of the goals of the European Union is to help citizens recognize the benefits of quieter, more

feller Foundation. theguardian.com/cities/2018/mar/08/where-world-noisiest-city.

peaceful spaces. To do that, the EU member countries have created an office within the Commission on Environment where questions of intrusive noise are taken seriously and addressed with clear guidelines and even some power of enforcement. It doesn't always work since much of the enforcement power is currently left to local authorities with ever-diminishing resources. (If Paris is an example of EU enforcement, then the policy's effectiveness might raise some sobering questions. But even Parisians noted with some surprise and relief how pleasantly quiet the city had become during the early stages of the COVID-19 lockdown.) Based on World Health Organization initiatives and working hand in hand with local jurisdictions, there have been several types of urban and suburban acoustic habitats trending to be more acoustically serene. In many European nations there is the collective will to find ways to dial down the noise. For example, the WHO guidelines for community noise recommend an ambient level of less than 30dB in bedrooms in order to get a good night's sleep. These are recommendations, not mandates. Enough citizens to make a difference are proactively aware of those guidelines and respectfully follow them.

To give you an idea of how quiet and relaxing that recommendation is, pick a time late at night or very early in the morning. Turn off the air conditioning, fans, washers and dryers, or forced air heat in your living space. Close all the doors and windows in and around your bedroom. Make sure the plumbing is quiet, and the fridge compressor is in standby mode. Check to see that no one has a TV or radio going in an adjacent room where the sound can penetrate the walls. No one should be snoring. Stand, breathing quietly in the middle of the room, and you'll get an idea how amazingly quiet and peaceful that moment can be. In fact, outside of bedrooms—like on the street—the nighttime sound level should be no greater than 40dB according to WHO objectives.

If we're hoping to create productive classroom environments, the ambient noise level should not be much louder than in a bedroom—only 35dB as a base measurement. Anything louder for sensitive young ears means increased levels of distraction, split attention, and escalated chances of learning disabilities. In a single solution almost universally overlooked, but one that bears repeating, the extent to which we cut the reverberation in classroom spaces down to less than three-tenths of a second, the reverence of learners within the space will increase demonstrably and the behavior of the young students will be much easier to address. Again, the psychological reason is simple: When children can't hear a reflection of their own voices, they tend to be much quieter, more focused, and respectful toward the environment and moment. There's also another benefit: Teachers aren't as exhausted by the end of the day. Everyone gains when the acoustic environment is well thought out and correctly implemented.

Most people affected by nighttime noise are children, who tend to be more sensitive to certain kinds of sounds than adults. The WHO report specifically addressed the side effects of noise on children—think of them as yours—and noted a high probability of impairment of early childhood development, an increase in learning disabilities and a number of lifelong effects on academic achievement and health. For example, studies on the effects of incessant childhood exposure to aircraft noise and constant near-field road traffic in the proximity of schools found that it weakened cognitive performance, as well as a sense of well-being and motivation, and indicated moderate levels of increased blood pressure and a hormone secretion that induced fight-or-flight responses.*

The elderly and chronically ill are also quite susceptible to disturbance, night or day, because they often sleep more lightly. Workers who change shifts frequently and whose sleep cycles are constantly being altered tend to be more stressed by noise that occurs during their resting phases for the same reason.

When you're deciding on an area that provides the best chances for sleep for you and your children, identify the quietest spaces and set up your bedrooms there. Consider also that the more sound-absorbent materials you place around the walls, floor, and windows, the more restful and tranquil your space will be at night. No matter what other factors may be at play in your life, a quiet, comfortable, safe spot to sleep can go a long way to making life less stressful and calm. All other things being equal, at the point when you are able to enjoy some decent and continuous nights of rest, you'll find

---

* Fritschi, Lin et al., *Burden of Disease From Environmental Noise: Quantification of Healthy Life Years Lose in Europe,* World Health Organization publication, March 2011.

yourself requiring fewer doctors' visits and won't have to rely on sleep meds.

Not incidentally, the WHO study goes on to report that about 40 percent of the population in the EU has been exposed to daytime road noise exceeding 55dB. Twenty percent have been subjected to daytime road noise levels exceeding 65dB. And more than 30 percent were affected by nighttime road noise that exceeded 55dB. While there is only a little international data on the direct health effects in the European region covered, early indicators suggest that they were far more positive than the conservative research teams had originally assumed. Based on anecdotal measurements, those EU-recommended numbers are considerably higher in most heavily populated American cities, although New York City has been addressing the issue for the past few years with neighborhood monitoring and the possibility of new restrictions.*

In the US, since the defunding of the Office of Noise Abatement, there are no recommended federal standards for noise levels. Enforcement rests with local law enforcement and most agencies have

---

* soundfighter.com/5-us-cities-with-the-highest-noise-levels/.

other priorities. Noise abatement is currently advocated by NGOs such as the Noise Pollution Clearing House.*

Now, ask yourself, if we did have a choice, why would any of us knowingly choose to live, work, or play in a place where we're susceptible to any kind of harmful condition? Without working models, or the collective will to modify our behavior, sometimes we haven't got many choices. When I got older, I was re-consigned to the noisiest part of my small childhood home, a corner room diagonally across from the old one, directly facing a busy street. There was no other option since my parents preferred the more quiet space. In addition to the issues I had to navigate with my ADHD, that move had a direct impact on my health and grades, both of which plummeted. My parents were not rich and couldn't afford a larger house in a neighborhood with houses set back from the street and more separation between them. At the time, from the late 1930s through the 1940s, double-paned windows to attenuate noise were not common or inexpensive. Few of us had the option of living outside cities in rural or wild areas where

_____
* https://www.nonoise.org.

there is less human-generated noise. Yet, according to the United Nations website, 54 percent [3.9 billion people] of the world's population now live in urban areas, a figure expected to increase to 66 percent as of 2050.* However, even with limited resources, we can go some distance in an effort to transform the habitats we do live in to make them more acoustically nourishing.

Since my noise irritant threshold is fairly low, in the last few decades there have been very few noise-free public urban settings that I've found to be comfortable, other than a few great concert halls in which I've either performed or attended as an audience member. That said, contemporary hotel structures, apartments, and home construction in large cities have improved to the point where interior atmospheres can be very soothing—as long as the heating and air-conditioning systems are quiet.

Our rammed earth home—the one that was destroyed by the fires—was a nearly perfect acoustic environment. With walls of earth two feet thick

---

* un.org/en/development/desa/news/population/world-urbanization -prospects-2014.html.

and recycled wood for the ceilings, the home was also eco-friendly and efficient to heat and cool. Because it was constructed of renewable materials (dirt from the site and recycled wood components) it was also a relatively inexpensive concept to build, especially where zoning laws are amenable. The color was a natural earth tone, so the surfaces never needed painting inside or out. And it turns out that the porous quality of the earthen walls naturally mediated the acoustics of the space like few other architectural solutions.

That reminds me of another use for the smartphone and iPad apps I mentioned earlier (see Physically Harmful Sounds—Chapter 2): You can measure these interior levels for yourself and see/hear how much noise there is where you live, work, and play. And this software is pretty accurate. Kat and I use these apps so we don't exceed our tolerance for stress in high-volume human habitats like sporting events, downtown streets at rush hour, restaurants, and entertainment venues. We've come to realize that all soundscapes affect our health, some of them in really good ways. Others, not. Either way, it is axiomatic that the quieter we are on the outside, the more peaceful we become inside.

Okay. I know what some of you are thinking: Where's the fun in all this? Two things to consider: No matter what your source of entertainment—specifically if it includes a loud audio component—make sure to protect your ears. Otherwise, you're doing to your ears the equivalent of what you do to your eyes if you were looking directly into the sun or a laser light. The second point: Leave yourself the space and time at the other extreme to find peaceful, undistracted moments. Tranquility has become a treasured commodity in these times, the most challenging that humans have encountered in a long while. If you value your mental and physical health, then this essential is probably at a similar level of priority as food, sleep, and regular exercise, again, assuming all things being equal. Draw on it frequently.

Bear in mind that there are many kinds of noises aside from those of an acoustic nature. There is visual noise made up of items demanding your attention, like ads in a magazine or pop-ups on your laptop or endless smartphone messages. There are the incessant reminders to stay connected via social media. There is the noise of light pollution in our cities blocking out the night skies. All of this makes for a field of noise in our lives that, because we allow it, never lets up. Stephen King, the author of *Cujo* and *The Shining,* recently quit Facebook because of the noise the platform brought into his life. Pico Iyer, the British-born essayist and novelist—in a recent *Quarantine Tapes* podcast—mentioned that he can only tolerate about five minutes of TV news because of the constant noise it produces with no useful information. If you want to feel connected and considered, pay a visit to a friend or supportive relative you feel close to, have a cup of tea or coffee, and just hang out, assuming the COVID protocols allow safe gatherings.

If you're traveling, there are many cities around the world that offer silent walks, eateries, and other facilities, some of them noted in publications such as *National Geographic* or *Lonely Planet Traveller.* Alaska is one of my favorite places to visit and record because it's a state three times the size of France with only about 730,000 residents. The territory features almost thirty-four thousand miles of Arctic, sub-Arctic, and northern temperate shoreline that includes temperate rain forests, boreal forests, tundra, mountain ranges, glaciers, estuaries, deltas, and hundreds of other habitats. Any one of them is extremely beautiful to visit, and many are remote enough that you might not hear another human-generated sound for days at a time.

For other tranquil places, Kat and I spent part of our honeymoon at the Monastery of Christ in the Desert, a magical desert location not far from Abiquiú, New Mexico, where dinners were eaten in silence and where the Benedictine monks had taken non-talking vows. If that's a bit too austere, there are wild, quiet habitats like this all over New Mexico where one can find true solace, and where the coyotes sing up the moon, and the cactus wrens, plovers, kingfishers, falcons, and ravens join a chorus of insects and frogs especially during the spring migration.

No matter where you live, there's likely a meditative open space nearby. We live about fifty miles north of the Golden Gate Bridge and San Francisco. Within a ninety-minute drive, I can find a dozen welcoming, quiet, and remote sites to chill without interruption for long periods.

In the late 1980s, Montana musician and friend Phil Aaberg and I traveled from Nogales, Arizona, on the US–Mexico border, following and recording the sounds of spring as it ranged north over the high-desert western landscape an average of forty-three miles a day. The route we decided upon was the 111 Meridian—also known by several Native American groups as "The Good Red Road"—a traditional vision quest corridor for many tribes. The course took us through the most spectacular parts of the American West—the Four Corners region, the Escalante, and the Wasatch range, past Yellowstone into the Bob Marshall Wilderness, all the way to the Canadian border just north of Chester, Montana.* Apart from Salt Lake City, the Western valley corridor of the Wasatch Mountains along I-15, and West Yellowstone, and with the exception of common domestic farm animals, we encountered relatively little disruptive noise along the back roads of that 1,400-mile two-month-long journey, giving us the ability to record almost the entire length of that route at most times of day or night. Those recordings served as the inspiration for our music and natural soundscape odyssey album, *Meridian*.

The objective with *Meridian* was to create our own sense of time and space—a reflection of our high desert encounters. You can do the same. With

---

* The Good Red Road is a path of discovery that is different for everyone. But the 111 Meridian was unique because individuals could truly abandon themselves to long periods of solitude anywhere within its vicinity.

sound, anything you can imagine that restores the soul is worth aiming for. If you want to try something fun and challenging, follow and record the route notably taken by Lewis and Clark from St. Louis all the way to the Pacific. It's a gorgeous course, and one not yet recorded in the way I and my colleagues like to do. If you're a history lover, as I am, just dreaming about that journey will make you wonder what all the fuss was about since Native Americans and First Nations people had already explored and populated North America along and far beyond that two-thousand-mile route many millennia before.

The spaces that heal

Check it out: When you enter a room or large space, close your eyes for a moment and consider how that habitat makes you feel based on your acoustic assessment. You really don't have to say anything or clap your hands. All of the sonic information is there. If the space makes you feel comfortable, all's well. If it doesn't, how would you go about fixing it, particularly if it meant that you'd be spending lots of time in that location?

CHAPTER 6

The Future Belongs to Those Who Can Hear It Coming

A paraphrase of David Bowie's aphorism spots a momentary position on our journey through the firmament. Meanwhile, back on Earth, amidst all the noise and fierce ambition, what remains to be heard?

The wolf's howl?

The blissful voice of ten thousand birds singing up the sun?

And where are the frogs and insects that signify a midsummer's night?

Whale-song in an open ocean?

The anxious declaration of an ant?

A virus liberating itself from a tiny cell?

No. It isn't music — the self-referential echo of our own limitations — that restores us.

It's a lone cricket awaiting an answer;

And our readiness to overhear the implications.

Even with eyes wide open, what is essential must first be heard.

José Emilio Pacheco is right: Night will never be night without the cricket.

Not to put too fine a point on it, but we've now reached the pinnacle of our acoustic pyramid. Superimpose the classic image of the all-seeing Eye of God or Providence watching over humanity and you get one perspective. Since we're talking about sound, let's change out the eye and drop in the image of an all-hearing ear. What nourishing signals will it detect as it seeks to repair the soundscape of the moment, given the course we've set for ourselves? What will it hear later today, or tomorrow, or next year? Does that emblematic ear detect healthy signs of life, wisdom, conciliation, kindness, love, wonder, beneficence, remedy, and restoration going forward? Or does it sense relentless strains of enmity, distortion, and signals more reminiscent of deep social affliction and spiritual depravity? What is it about Bowie's aphorism, the title of this chapter, that seems so prescient? None of this really hits home until our all-hearing ear senses the kind of tranquility we must have within range in order to thrive. It needs to be a clear objective, one that can be attained when we desire a moment and the space to restore our body and mind to positive states of being.

The most remarkable feature of the COVID-19 pandemic is the surprising responses Kat and I received from friends, colleagues, and even strangers reaching out from across the globe calling attention to the incredible variety of sonic anecdotes I've been referring to. With so many layers of noise reduced or eliminated during the first months of the lockdown, our astute ear detected sounds of spring 2020 present and accounted for in locations never anticipated and in ways never before heard in the lifetimes of many adults no matter where they lived. One of my book editors wrote about having morning coffee on his fire escape outside his apartment in Carroll Gardens, Brooklyn, listening to urban birds sing and feeling a deep sense of wonder at the spectacle because he'd never heard that soundscape before. A cheery observation in these otherwise dark times. Another writes: "Now that I am older...I find sleeping harder to come by. These [soundscapes]

really helped me relax...I think part of my motivation is...surgery next week, and that's not much
fun recovering from, so I hope these soundscapes
relax me—in a good way." And there are some indi-
cations that stress itself may increase our vulnerabil-
ity to viral infection. This certainly holds true for
the hardy wood frog.* If I'm any example, natural
soundscapes introduced into our personal spaces
help reduce that stress.

A colleague in Munich reported that his kids
played on the patio outside their house—their masks
on and minding social distances—reading to each
other and listening to the sounds of spring, noting
for the first time in their young lives the unique song
each species of bird expressed and creating a game
out of the experience. Even though it's wintertime
in the southern hemisphere, a South African safari
guide remarked that wild animals are revealing
themselves more frequently. Emboldened by a land
freed from a glut of tourist vehicles that during "the
season" gives the plains a sense of rush-hour traffic density not unlike that in Times Square, wildlife

---

* phys.org/news/2020-05-amphibian-stress-vulnerability-virus.htm
l?MessageRunDetailID=1783930315&PostID=14608773&utm
_medium=email&utm_source=rasa_io.

temporarily fills the open spaces. Meanwhile, wild sound was coming from everywhere as birds, frogs, and mammals repopulated urban spaces with their subtle voices in habitats that humans had been obliged to forsake for weeks and, in some cases, months on end, for their own survival.

Being confined, as we were, during the pandemic, amplified by the effects of chronic ADHD and PTSD from the consequences of the 2017 Northern California fires that upended us, left some pretty sobering scars. With the combination of all these events in such a short period, depression and feelings of hopelessness became more difficult for us to manage. I began writing this piece before the COVID-19 event challenged all of my ideas about what a "normal" life meant. Given the instability of our population and the powerlessness of some of the human institutions we've created, with conditions amplified by the destructive leaders we've elected, I was clearly mistaken to embrace the illusion of more considered outcomes.

I have never been lonely. Not with Kat nearby— the most magnanimous loving person I've ever known. Hers is an openhandedness that takes my breath away. Yet, with my own demons to contend with, I'm reminded when all else fails of how often I turn to natural sound to help abate feelings of disconnection and anger and to enable a progression to something larger and more gratifying. Integral to those narrative signals is a sympathetic well that we all need to draw from in order to implement those outcomes.*

The most hopeful feedback I get usually comes from children. The kids from South Korea, to whom we introduced *The Great Animal Orchestra* performance piece in 2018, recounted their own experiences of the soundscapes in the exhibit that the Fondation Cartier, United Visual Artists (UVA, London), and I installed in Seoul. Their enthusiasm reminded me of my own encouraging words to stay alert for the good things that result from all that's occurring around us. These global reminders coalesce in the way biophonies animate a sense of the living world. By doing so the youngsters reassure those of us who care that they are already thinking of their future, one that embraces a thriving planet of wildlife. "What kind of sound does a whale make?" asks

---

* I'll take the anthropomorphic criticism here. For the doubters, my morph is definitely anthropophic.

one child—one of her first attempts toward links with The Other.*

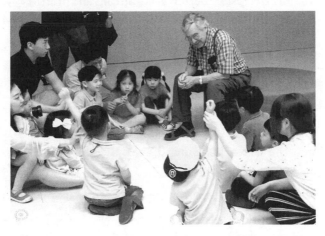

Seoul Museum of Art and the *Great Animal Orchestra* workshop with soundscape ecologist Bernie Krause.

Friends and colleagues alike, taking short breaks from the virus's confinement, walk the streets of cities, large and small, hearing urban wildlife unconstrained for the first time. From their descriptions, most don't miss the harmful noise that continually bore down on them in the old, "normal" days that

---

* https://www.fondationcartier.com/en/exhibitions/le-grand-orchestre -des-animaux.

abruptly ended in mid-March 2020. With some, whose lives haven't been infected by more virulent cultural diseases, better possibilities abound. How can you be distressed when you hear the graceful song of a bird reestablishing its rightful territory knowing that a nest and clutch of eggs can't be far behind?

Where Kat and I were living temporarily in the midst of a Northern California vineyard after the fires, the dawn birdsong during the spring of 2020 was rich with many different variants. Recordings I made then conferred my own account of a natural resurrection on Easter Sunday. That's the congregation I joined long ago and the one I rejoice with most of the time. There's no thought or need for social distancing there. Masks don't matter. The sermon comes to you directly from the heart and soul of the universe. It's as organic, potent, and as spiritual as it gets.

Paper after paper, email after email, and an endless stream of letters convey the impression that if we just leave things alone, without the compulsion to intercede and "fix" everything, restoration occurs. Immediately after the lockdown was initiated, much of the toxic haze that blanketed most major cities in the world dissipated as satellite images so persuasively illustrated. Wildlife that had never been seen before appeared in our neighborhoods, to the delight of kids and adults all of whom marveled at the sound the animal orchestra produced through the lively choruses of these organisms. With the cessation of commercial traffic, the canal water in Venice, Italy, was clear enough to see fish for the first time in memory. Whale vocalizations could be picked up sixty miles away in oceans that had quieted down with much of the large vessel noise gone. All we needed to do was to *stop* moving, consuming, competing, driving, and shouting about our presence. Some of us did that and noted the difference. We took a badly needed but involuntary rare breath of fresh air. Unfortunately, all too many weren't paying attention and soon lost patience.

Here's a description that I received at the end of April from a friend living in Italy: "It's a strange time. Happily, the sounds of nature have been amplified, if such can be said, and the traffic noise was almost gone. We've been in total lockdown for almost three months. Yesterday the governor of

Liguria loosened the restrictions. We're of two minds about this. Already, the noise level has gone up, people are flowing back into the panoramic *passeggiata* (promenade) that snakes from San Rocco past the house...bringing human noises, dog noises, telephone noises...not to mention coughs and sneezes and worse."

Even so, one of the best choices you can make is to spend quality time outside. Go to a park if there are no larger green spaces nearby. Most of these are free, open spaces. If you have access to a larger forested area, even better. And do it with safety in mind, at off-peak hours when there's not so much city noise. Don't talk. Just walk slowly and listen. Every season, no matter where you live, speaks to you through its special biophony. I can't emphasize enough how important it is to connect to a natural world experience in order to become more conscious of the quality of spaces you'll want to live in. Expressions of those tranquil natural surroundings are situated in that vast life-sustaining domain, waiting for you to pick and choose among them. Hearing is believing. And belief changes everything.

Other than the joy of being outdoors, there are two healthful features to keep in mind as goals: One is the quality of your living space. The other relates to the types of soundscapes you choose to fill that biome with.

Perhaps crisis encounters are the kinds of events we need in order to oblige positive changes in our lives. It's that kick in the ass that restrains us from more obsessive behavior where the limits of our control delusion have finally been reached. In the end, we're going to have to figure out how to switch out the encounters that harm us with nourishing actions that sustain. Whole communities benefit if the choices we make as individuals and family groups are conscious, and not knee-jerk reactions to disaster, crises, and fantasy. While the soundscapes with which we choose to surround ourselves are good places to begin, no particular acoustic space or recorded natural sound will help much if the overall mindset of the culture fails to move proactively in support of less stressful and less destructive social, cultural, and environmental behavior. We've reached a time in our saga when, if we intend to thrive, we have no other choice.

Bernie Krause

Things to do, now:

1. Heed the narratives expressed through the biophony. Our history is writ large within those stories.
2. Be quiet.
3. Listen.
4. Be amazed.

Epilogue of *Sons Disparus* (Disappeared Sounds) and Those Returning for One Last Plea to Flourish

The biophonies of Aceh Province in Sumatra have changed markedly since the tragic tsunami events of late December 2004. The forest is quiet whether by changes within the landscape or because many of the animals have fled elsewhere. Possibly it's a combination of both issues. Humans, needing fuel to cook with and wood to build their dwellings, have tapped into forest resources accessible to them for those essentials. The population needs the wood, but they rely on the sounds of the forest, as well. It's a dilemma that has no easy resolution. I glance sadly at pre-fire pictures of the DAT tapes marked "Sumatra" sitting on a shelf in my old lab and wonder if a long silent period will finally descend there as it has in so many other locations. I do not handle these moments very well and know that I am not alone.

Elders in the Wyam tribe tell of a time that they fished all year long at Celilo Falls, a little Native American community west of the Columbia River's midway point. Each season provided lots of fish including Chinook salmon, bluebacks, steelhead, and coho. When the catch was good, members could harvest a ton of fish a day—soon having enough to supply close and extended family all that was needed for a year with little more than the cost of a couple of balls of twine. In recent history a major event took place along the Columbia River in the Pacific Northwest. It went unnoticed by most of the media, but it profoundly affected those who had lived in the region for thousands of years.

On the morning of March 10, 1957, the Army Corps of Engineers ordered the massive steel gates of the newly built Dalles Dam shut tight. This action strangled the natural downstream flow of the river. As the Elders stood on the riverbank astonished, a way of life that had sustained them for centuries disappeared in less than a day. It all happened very quickly. Six hours later and eight miles upstream, the sacred falls of the Wyam were completely submerged. That day there wasn't a dry eye on the banks near Celilo, that tiny village on the river's edge. The Elders were not weeping for the loss of salmon. They wept because the river no longer lent its wise voice to the community. The submerged Celilo Falls were dead silent. Members report that with the loss of their natural music, the tribe was plunged into a deeper collective despair than at any time since contact with whites.

April 1, 2020, Sonoma, California, after three weeks of COVID shutdown and almost no automobile traffic. The clear-aired view from the hillside on which our postfire temporary living space is located extends forty miles. We can see detail in the high-rise buildings of downtown San Francisco forty miles to our south.* Our little valley is quiet now, and we hear birds and insects during times they were not previously audible.

April 13, 2020. Kat and I stepped outside early to drink our morning coffee and, already, the bright

_____

* Caveat: npr.org/sections/health-shots/2020/05/19/854760999/traffic-is-way-down-due-to-lockdowns-but-air-pollution-not-so-much.

blue skies were again cross-stitched with the contrails of jets. Two weeks ago that view was completely clear.

April 15, 2020. The dawn chorus at nearby Sugarloaf Ridge State Park is spectacular today. But something's changed. The usual mix of birdsong, present for nearly a decade beginning in the early 1990s, is gone. It has been replaced with a new chorus of singers that have recently appeared. It's not just the virus. It's probably also due to the fact that we're nine years into a historic drought that brought with it massive fires, the burns so intense that they wiped out whole communities including this one for the second time in three years. Spring now begins two weeks earlier than it did in any year of the 1990 decade. With the shifting migration patterns, I don't recognize the soundscape any longer, everything is so different. It sets me on edge to hear the scale of the transformation.

May 12, 2020. Way too early, the government, under pressure from industry, has begun to open up California for business. Downtown San Francisco, forty miles distant on the horizon, is no longer visible from our hillside—the view gone in just a few days as we find ourselves slouching toward "normal." Automobile traffic has increased, and I hear the persistent whoosh of human mobility drowning out the full-throated song of a mockingbird perched at the apex of a lodgepole pine nearby.

The confusing passive-aggressive acoustic environment created by the TV news is mostly noise—self-justifying and incomprehensible. I return to it after a three-year hiatus only to find that it still gives me nothing of value but a headache and indigestion. Because of the ways in which the cable and regular networks frame their presentations, mostly as carriers for elder-related medicinal ads, the few minutes of compressed information that we do get tend to be more confusing than informative or helpful. Nevertheless, if we can only discern tiny grains of truth, we might learn how to transform them into useful templates. We just have to remember that facts are not truth. The truth is what you do with facts.

"People are dying…and all you can talk about is money! How dare you!" warned Greta Thunberg during her impassioned UN Climate Summit presentation in September 2019. Like Ms. Thunberg, most climate-literate people realize that every financial model depends, ultimately, on access to natural resources. Unless we stop and reconsider the consequences of plundering those finite repositories, we will—if we haven't already—find ourselves beyond a point of no return where key reserves have been depleted beyond any chance of restoration. The impoverishment we've unleashed on humanity and the rest of the living world is conveyed through the narratives of the biophony. And it correlates directly with the obsessive levels of anxiety and fear that are ripping apart the living fabric of this planet, not to mention the human social one. Thunberg urges us to find inspired ways to change those pernicious behavioral patterns and instead embrace those more compatible and life-affirming actions sooner rather than later. If she and we can help others realize the wisdom of this action, our chances might still be good. After all, her mission has centered and helped to restore her, as mine has me. But right now, every sign at this crossroad of choices points to "critical."

As this pandemic crisis reveals all too clearly, we're a lonely, obsessive culture. Vulnerable and needy.

Many of us have a hard time flying solo for any period. Luckily, I've found comfort in solitude because of the nature of my work and because my type of ADHD keeps me creatively occupied. When in the presence of The Others (the nonhuman animal world) that I'm listening to or recording, I feel intimately connected. To some, loneliness and isolation are terrifying. But my fieldwork has seriously challenged that paradigm. I have to work alone both in the field (if I don't want the continuity of my recordings compromised by the noise I or others bring along), but also in the studio when I'm creating sonic works of art. Those moments, basking in the soft voices of the natural world, are the resonances I need to hear in order to feel centered and linked to something larger. For me, the forest, desert, and ocean biophonies are the voices of the divine, the sermons from the mount, the spiritual homilies of ancient times, and as the late naturalist and author Paul Shepard suggested: a spot in the Pleistocene from which we've never departed.

Natural mimics, we learned the roots of our music, language, and movement from the creature voices of the natural world, as we tend to copy the signatures that currently surround us. When you become familiar and comfortable with them, they'll tend to burrow deep into your soul. It bears repeating that elements of these biophonies that engage us may even be rooted within our DNA. To our unfortunate loss, though, the acoustic impressions that now dominate are composed primarily of noise, elements we try to overcome with yet more competing noise, some of it framed as sound art. We need to take care in our constant struggle to separate noise from useful signal, lest we misread important information that comes our way. It's evident in many forms. For example, the ways in which we hear the messages of those we disagree with as useless sound are often echoed back to us as mockery or disdain. What do we signify that inspires that reaction? How do we change that model?

The narrative that signals physical and emotional states of a wild habitat is expressed eloquently through the voice of the natural world, its biophony. When I'm a bit under the weather, as with a cold, that disorder shows in my voice. It's the same with the collective voices of the wild. Affect a thriving habitat of living organisms by resource extraction, pollution, noise, or land transformation, and you'll clearly know by its sound how radically we've altered it. More often than not, these days our behavior and the critter responses are not positive. Only we can alleviate that problem. Every path to the remedies achieved through tranquility is up to us; and only we can harness the resources and the will to ensure the necessary restorative action.

In this last phase of life my remaining energies are dedicated to sharing my insights with you and with folks across all cultures and ages through my work in the fine arts. My goal here is to somehow transform esoteric concepts into feelings much more tangible and accessible. Through this lens I aim to convey how the power of sound furnishes perception into the rest of the living world and illuminates our deep links to it. Each of us in our own way has to become still and listen again if the heartbeat of this planet and the life-forms that sustain it are to be heard and thrive. As for the flip side of that coin, it is pretty clear that the further we remove ourselves from our primary connection to the natural world the more pathological our behavior becomes. We are beginning to inhabit a world where crises of the kinds we incurred during the pandemic of 2020 will likely occur with more frequency, each one accompanied with its own unique soundtrack. Before the next one strikes, and it will, allow yourself a few minutes each day to meditate on the few changes each one of us must make to restore the means to love again. It'll be the best soundtrack you'll ever hear.

Sharing this message is a two-pronged strike involving science, on the one hand, and art on the other. With science, we stick to abstract protocols to explain the observable outcomes of our work. The interpretation of these data and their consequences serve as the basis for how we then present our case to colleagues and in professional forums. In the arts, however, we focus on the emotional impact of the subject, while at the same time maintaining the integrity of the topic. From my own perspective and my own large-scale works, I show how the power of sound illustrates what occurs in an abruptly changing ecosphere. All of the proofs are there—just in a different form not often considered before. My idea of art is to create performances of wonder I most want others to hear and see manifest in the world.

Supplemental Summary — To Do List

1. **What to listen to. What to listen for.**
2. **The sound walk**
   a. Name all of the sounds you hear (and know) in the soundscape
      i. What do the sounds you recognize mean to you?
      ii. Are the sounds you DON'T recognize meaningful?
   b. What sounds do you like?
      i. Why?
      ii. What are the specific qualities that appeal to you?
   c. What sounds bother you?
      i. Why?
      ii. How would you alter those elements (if you could)?

d. Describe your ideal soundscape—the one that you would choose to surround you most of the time.

3. Sound and noise—distinguish between "signal" and "noise."

1. **Sound walk 1**—walk outside anywhere in your neighborhood and note on paper the different types of sound you hear. In any soundscape, there are typically three basic sources.
   a. Which do you like and why?
   b. Which bother you and why?

2. **Sound walk 2**—walk in the woods (or any other habitat) for the pure joy of it. Ask the same questions as Sound walk 1 (above).

3. **Apps**—for $.99 you can download sound level apps. Learn to use them to find comfortable spaces for yourself. Keep in mind that it's not always the level that matters, but the quality of the sound source and the habitat in which it's heard. In the latter case, rely on your ears and what they tell you.
   a. Is the soundscape of the habitat you're in relaxing?

b. Is the soundscape of the habitat you're in stressful?

c. What are the qualities that convey those conditions?

4. **If you prefer to listen to music or podcast programs with earbuds,** keep the levels down. If you have to crank them to hear the detail in a noisy environment, move to a more tranquil spot to listen. Be sure you can still hear enough of the world beyond the earbuds to stay alert to your surroundings.

5. **Create a safe, acoustically serene place—one without reverberation—where you live so that...**

a. you can sleep undisturbed by extraneous noise.

b. you can be engaged in ways that energize you.

c. you feel less stressed.

6. **Record or download soundscapes that make you feel good.**

a. Begin experimenting with your smartphone. If you like what you hear and want to go further...

b. Pick up a digital recorder (Zoom H4n, Sony, Panasonic, smartphone, etc.) and try those for a while. You can find that tech for under $200. Any of those devices should provide what you need until you want to move to professional-level equipment. It took me ten years to learn to record the sound of ocean waves so they sounded right when played back in a room with speakers. Have patience. It's really fun and will help you learn to listen as you focus on acoustic subjects to capture. The textures and wonders are endless.

7. Fill your unique acoustic space with sounds that soothe, fascinate, and enrich your life. Imaginings—what would you hear if...

A. you were a bat?
B. you were a cat?
C. you were an elephant?
D. you were a dog?

8. **Listen!**

Acknowledgments

There are five people I acknowledge here, without whose help and support this book would not have been written. The first is my agent, Gillian MacKenzie, who orchestrated the opportunity and refused to let me submit anything other than what we proposed. The second is my dear wife and partner, Kat, who, during this process, cleared an emotional path for me and us as we continue our recovery from the Northern California fires that wiped us out in 2017, the fires that threatened us in 2018 and 2019 that didn't, but whose effects we still feel every time a dry, hot wind comes up from the East. Then there is Professor Kevin Padian, Evolutionary Biologist from UC Berkeley and dear friend, whose narrative map is writ large over every page. And finally, my editors, Phil Marino, who helped organize this chronicle of an otherwise obscure and elusive subject, and Elizabeth Gassman, who set the lyrics to a proper cadence.

Bernie Krause

*   *   *

This book is dedicated to the late Stuart Gage, Professor Emeritus, Michigan State University, who championed the concepts of geophony, biophony, and anthropophony, the acoustic niche hypothesis (ANH), and the nascent field of Soundscape Ecology, when no one else heard the orchestration. And special kudos to Al Young, longtime friend and mentor, California Poet Laureate, whose own poetry and stories long ago inspired my pursuit of the written word.

About the Author

Dr. Bernie Krause is a former composer and musician. He is an author, naturalist, and artist exploring the world of soundscape ecology, bioacoustics, and natural sound. In 1968, he founded Wild Sanctuary, an organization dedicated to the recording and archiving of natural soundscapes.